Malaria
The Evolution of a Killer

Norma Mohr

SERIF & PIXEL

Serif & Pixel Press

Seattle

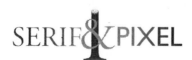

Serif & Pixel Press

770 North 34th Street

Seattle, WA 98103

www.booksatoz.com

Cover and book design by Books AtoZ

ISBN 0-9713872-0-6

Printed in the United States of America

First printing, 2001

Dedication

This book is dedicated to many individuals:

First, to my late husband Charley Mohr, who will always enrich my memories.

Then, to our children and grandchildren, who carry his warmth and sparkle. I am deeply grateful to them all and pray that my work does them justice.

I would be remiss if I did not also acknowledge my gratitude for the impeccable editorial assistance provided by Babak Emami.

Table of Contents

PART I
MALARIA IN THE UNITED STATES

Chapter 1: Modern times
Malaria was always a good traveler. Even in modern times California was an open door for the disease.

Chapter 2: A land of opportunity
War and migrations are bad for the health. Southern doctors create control strategies.

Chapter 3: Creeping prosperity
Mississippi Basin, Cuba and Panama attract the disease, but recovery is fast.

Chapter 4: Golden age of malariology
Public health strategies are born from the Great Depression and DDT.

PART II
THE PARASITE AND ITS UNIVERSE

Chapter 5: The lifestyle of the parasite
The parasite and the human immune system compete for survival.

Chapter 6: World history
Ancient Greece, a cure from Peru and two World Wars.

Chapter 7: The malaria vaccine

A malaria vaccine? Not yet. Some folks give up.

Chapter 8: New paths, old paths

A breakthrough cure? Not yet.

PART III
MALARIA IN THE DEVELOPING WORLD

Chapter 9: Sub-Saharan Africa
Africa suffers the most malaria, by far. There must be a reason.

Chapter 10: Southeast Asia

In Southeast Asia, war connives with malaria. Highland forests have old aggressive strains.

Chapter 11: Fire in the Amazon

Amazon's epidemic, worst in history. Public health policies hold it back.

Introduction to the Author

Norma Mohr is a retired American journalist who grew up along Chicago's northern reaches. Her parents and other family members were writers. She remembers, "I assumed that's what you do when you grow up."

In her early career she worked as a dictation typist for the Washington Bureau of the Associated Press, then as a writer for the *Washington Post*, and finally as a writer/copy editor for the United Press Bureau in Chicago.

In 1960 she and her husband, Charles Mohr of the *New York Times* moved overseas for 15 years. They lived in India, Hong Kong, Thailand and Kenya. While Charles was staff correspondent for the *New York Times* and *Time* Magazine, Norma reared their four children, studied languages and wrote freelance articles.

It was then that she acquired a deep sympathy for the destitute women and children of the so-called Third World. Many of them were homeless, living in the streets at the fringes of town, or at the open-air markets outside of town, clustered around a solitary tamarind tree. Many of those young children wore charms from local healers for protection from malaria and other diseases. The babies had protruding stomachs indicating malnutrition. Flies crowded around their listless eyes. The common scene always filled Mohr with profound grief. But she was comforted by her promise to herself to find a way to help them.

When Mohr and her family moved back to the U.S., she took a succession of jobs: editor for the Audubon Naturalist Society; editor and writer for the Office for Civil Rights, Department of Health, Education, and Welfare; and finally as a senior editor with the Voice of America — the U.S. agency that broadcasts overseas.

That was where Mohr saw her first opportunity to fulfill her solemn promise to help the women of the developing world. She was assigned to collaborate with foreign broadcasters, health providers, and officials of Health Ministries from several developing countries to create special programs. The result was a weekly radio series for women who rarely, if ever, could receive professional health care. The series, called "Your Healthy Family," was translated and broadcast in 40 languages in the developing world.

The programs consisted of scripted dialogues between a fictitious health care worker — "Sister Hawa" — and a mother with lots of health-related questions. Topics were chosen with great care and included issues seldom discussed on the radio. Mohr said she tried to address what she called real needs. Several African physicians and radio announcers helped her, including Dr. Gladys Hadiza George-Diolombi, a Nigerian physician trained in Sweden. The two, Mohr and George, met at Mohr's office every Sunday to choose topics and to draft scripts. They talked about:

- How to prepare for the arrival of the birth attendant;
- How to keep the house ventilated to protect the new baby's lungs;
- How to build a litter for transporting a sick person to the nearest clinic;
- How to take care of an invalid at home;

- How to plan a vegetable garden to protect children against malnutrition, and more.

One Sunday Dr. George was exceptionally excited. She rushed into Mohr's office, saying "You wouldn't believe what I just learned." She had attended a lecture by a physician from Singapore who told his audience how to protect themselves against malaria. For example, they could join forces with their neighbors in altering their environment to prevent mosquitoes from breeding near their homes. Sometimes all that was needed to stop malaria was a neighborhood campaign to alter the course of a stream. Other times, just uprooting young trees and bushes that sheltered a pool and attracted mosquitoes was adequate. It was surprising to Dr. George to learn that such small projects could transform an unhealthy environment into a safe one.

Each project represented what public health specialists referred to as "sanitary engineering." It's a branch of civil engineering concerned primarily with the maintenance of environmental conditions conducive to public health. George said, "Why didn't they teach us that in Sweden!" In fact, most medical schools in those days overlooked the basic maintenance of public health in deference to highly technical strategies. The collaborations with Dr. George and others inspired Mohr to seek a way to illuminate the story about malaria and its prevention. That's how this book was born.

After the death of her husband in 1989, Mohr retired from the Voice of America and moved to Seattle where she eventually completed work on her malaria book. During the same period she also became cofounder and then President of the Greater Seattle Vietnam Association. She and her colleagues there established a sister-city relationship between Seattle and Haiphong, Vietnam. Her concern for the health of women and children followed her everywhere.

Part I

Malaria in the United States

A friend said, "Do you really think anyone in the U.S. is interested in malaria?" My answer was "Yes." No other disease has left such a mark on humankind. Malaria was intertwined in the culture and history of people everywhere. It was common in the U.S. from precolonial times until about 1875. The disease continued to threaten Americans until the late 1930s.

N.M.

Eleven days after returning from Africa, a 59-year-old Illinois woman went to a local hospital complaining of fever, chills, body aches and shortness of breath. The woman had just returned from a 6-week missionary trip to Kenya and Zaire. She wasn't able to recall if she had taken any antimalarial medicine. Upon admission to the hospital, the initial laboratory studies revealed few blood platelets and evidence of kidney failure. She developed respiratory distress and was transferred to the intensive-care unit of a referral hospital where she was put on an artificial kidney machine. A microscopic analysis of her blood revealed the presence of falciparum malaria infection. More than 5% of her red blood cells contained malaria parasites. Treatment with intravenous quinidine was initiated. Despite her treatment, the woman continued to deteriorate. The following day, she was dead.
(Malaria Surveillance – United States, 1995; MMWR 48 (SS-1): 1–23, 1999).

Chapter 1
Modern Times

Y ES, EVEN IN THE 1990s Americans were still dying of malaria, known as history's worst disease. The worldwide toll was growing, taking millions of human casualties in the developing world and threatening other people who traveled there. In fact, according to some specialists, more people were dying of malaria throughout the world than ever before (BBC Online, 1998). Experts believed the situation was getting worse (Najera, 1992). In regions where malaria was firmly entrenched, most individuals over five years of age had acquired a partial immunity to the parasite. They were at least a little sick most of the time, but they were safe from full-blown malaria as long as they got reinfected intermittently. Children under five had insufficient immunity and the highest death rate by far. According to a prominent U.S. malariologist, it was estimated that 10,000 children died every single day of malaria worldwide (Steve Hoffman on BBC Online, 1998).

A tourist in a highly malarious region was like a nonimmune baby whose first infection could kill him. Doctors believed that only 30 to 60 percent of malaria infections imported into the U.S. were reported to health authorities. There were several reasons.

At first, the typical victim might believe he was just suffering from the flu. Perhaps the family doctor came to the same conclusion. Most U.S. physicians didn't see enough malaria to recognize it initially. It would help if the patient told the doctor about that recent trip to the tropics, but an individual with bad malaria was usually disoriented. Maybe he forgot about the trip. Maybe he had felt at the time that he was perfectly safe from malaria because he took the best preventive medicine available. It was becoming clear that the best preventive medicine available simply was not good enough.

Many individuals who took drugs to prevent the infection were getting malaria from the ever-emerging, virulent, drug - resistant strains. Finally, when the "flu" kept getting worse, diagnostic blood tests might be performed. But often the technicians didn't know what to look for. That is, they might not recognize the malaria parasites in the blood smears. To make it even harder, parasites of the *falciparum* species[1], the worst kind of malaria, often sequestered themselves in the tissues of the human host, and they were not immediately visible through a microscope (Cook, 1989; Greenberg, 1990; Freedman, 1992; Miller, 1989).

Old Medications Lose Power

Travelers and members of the armed forces remembered when the threat of malaria was minimal, and protection against the disease was routine and reliable. An individual just took some tablets before leaving for the tropics, continued the medication while away and then kept up with the same pills for another few weeks after returning home.

It used to be rare indeed for the disease to break through that protection. Mosquitoes might still bite and might inject malaria parasites in the person's blood, but the organisms usually did not survive long enough or in great enough numbers to cause serious illness.

There used to be two good medicines that people could rely on: quinine and chloroquine. Quinine was made from the bark of a South American tree and used to be effective against malaria. But in order to cure malaria with quinine one had to take large doses of it for long periods of time. When quinine became less and less effective against malaria, chloroquine took its place.

Chloroquine was a wonderful drug. It was cheap, easy to tolerate even in young children and very effective. It worked against both common types of the disease: vivax and falciparum malaria. Many years later it was still effective against vivax malaria. But during the 1960s falciparum malaria began to show signs of resistance to the drug, just the way some other diseases were developing resistance to widely used antibiotics. Consequently, medicines that used to cure or prevent the disease no longer worked. Then *P. falciparum* quickly acquired resistance to many subsequent drugs created to replace chloroquine.

By the 1980s there were many antimalarial drugs on the market but no clear choice for use worldwide. It was confusing for tourists, especially when they had a chance to compare advice with one another.

That happened for instance when a group of eight American women friends met for a long-awaited camel safari in northern Kenya in 1988. On the first night, eight cots were laid out beside the river, with a mosquito net hanging over each one. As night fell and the women lingered around the campfire, they compared what each had been told about malaria by their doctors back in the US or in Britain. Each of the eight was given a different regimen of medicine for preventing malaria. No two of them had the same advice (Author, 1988).

One survey showed that between 1985 and 1991 more than 80 different drug regimens were used by travelers in Kenya (Steffen, 1993). It was not that so many effective medicines were

5

available. The fact was, there was no longer one that was generally recognized as a completely safe and reliable choice. New medicines kept appearing, and old medicines were resurrected. Combinations of the new and the old were tried.

Medicines that reportedly protected a traveler from malaria in one country or region were unreliable in another, and the picture kept changing as drug-resistant strains of the disease seemed to creep from region to region (Hall, 1992; Freedman, 1992).

Besides the problem of efficacy, many of the new medicines carried at least some risk of side effects in doses strong enough to cure an established infection. After all, an antimalarial medicine must be toxic enough to kill millions or billions of live microscopic parasites. One of the new drugs was found to be unsafe for pregnant women. Some doctors were recommending that pregnant women postpone their plans to travel to Africa, if possible. Families were advised not to take their babies or young children to malarious areas of Africa (Hall, 1992; Barry, 1992).

As malaria's resistance to medicines continued to spread, some travelers and some doctors were not counting on prophylactic or preventive medicine alone for protection. They turned to old practical precautions that were reliable before the era of "wonder drugs." One doctor said, "the old ways to prevent malaria are new again" (Sampaio, 1990). People living in malarious regions were taking steps to remove mosquito breeding areas from around their houses. That usually was not hard.

Tourists and other visitors were learning some of the old tricks. Many were having dinner in the hotel's indoor dining room instead of on the terrace, wearing long sleeved shirts and full length slacks, and applying mosquito repellent on exposed areas of their skin, especially the ankles. Some tourists were spraying insect repellent at the corners of their hotel bedroom at night. In hotels or lodges where the air conditioning may have broken down and the windows were left open, experienced travelers were insisting on mosquito nets and were making certain the nets were securely tucked in under the mattress (Lobel, 1989; Conlon, 1990; Hall, 1992).

For travelers who wanted preventive drugs as well as those old-fashioned practical precautions against being bitten, doctors with experience with malaria stressed the importance of having up-to-date advice before buying any medicine. Advice in a book or magazine or the media would not necessarily be valid. The same could be said about advice from a friend or the average general practitioner. Parasites rapidly and unpredictably altered their distribution and versatile defense strategies.[2] In many regions, mosquitoes that transported the disease were often changing their life-styles and their susceptibility to various drugs.

Individuals planning a trip and their doctors could get up-to-date advice from the U.S. Centers for Disease Control (CDC) or other similar agencies in other countries. Those agencies provided a public information telephone service giving details about which drugs were no longer effective or safe and details about specific regional conditions. Incidentally, CDC was the US public health agency created in 1946 for the purpose of fighting malaria.

By the end of the 20th century, most experts were assuming there was no perfect malaria medicine and probably never would be. Travelers headed for the tropics, regardless of the preventive measures they took, were advised to carry along additional or stronger medicine to take if they came down with symptoms of malaria before they got home. The person who treated the infection immediately, even with a less than perfect medicine, might reduce the risk of life-threatening complications. Those grave, potentially fatal complications often struck fast, appearing two to three hours after the onset of symptoms. Death could follow in a matter of days.

Malaria Flies to Great Britain

The United States was not the only prosperous and industrialized country threatened by its rising toll of malaria. In the Great Britain an upswing of imported malaria starting in the late 1970s followed the same pattern as in the United States, a pattern synchronized with the expanding distribution and virulence of the disease in the developing world.

By the early 1990s, the annual rate of imported malaria in Britain was about 2,000 cases. In the 10-year period ending in 1989, the numbers had risen 51 percent (Conlon, 1990). The total recorded for the U.S. in the early 1990s was 1,100, reflecting a comparable 10-year rise.

The higher number for Britain was due to the fact that a larger percentage of British residents traveled to Africa and Asia. They included people of African and Asian descent who had immigrated to Britain or had come to Britain to go to school. When they returned to their homelands for a visit, they risked coming back to Britain with malaria. Britain had a long ac-quaint-ance with malaria. Imagine all the British people who must have died of malaria, exploring, conquering and then ruling their far-flung colonies. Malaria never set on the British Empire.

The largest numbers of malaria carriers entering Great Britain in modern times were people who visited the Indian sub-continent and returned with vivax malaria or people who went to West Africa and returned with falciparum malaria. About 2 percent of the travelers returning from Ghana and 1 percent returning from Nigeria brought falciparum malaria with them. Of the total number of malaria cases imported into Britain in a 10-year period, the number attributed to falciparum malaria rose from 20 to 50 percent. Doctors in Great Britain expected the steady climb of imported falciparum malaria would continue (Bradley, 1989).

Health authorities throughout Britain responded to each new case on an emergency basis and assumed none of the imported malaria had spread. In fact, they believed that people who stayed home were more likely to get malaria from infected mosqui-toes that stowed away on airplanes from the tropics. More likely from stowaway mosquitoes, that is, than from infected ticketed

8

travelers. Infected people got quick attention. Infected mosquitoes, on the other hand, could just fly away.

London, as well as other European cities with international airports, suffered from a category of disease known to public health workers as "Airport Malaria" or "Airplane Malaria" or "Runway Malaria." African mosquitoes were already notorious for stowing away on ships and trucks, spreading disease as they went. In the 1970s, they were boarding wide-bodied jetliners parked on the runways of African airports. Sometimes mosquitoes invaded the interiors of the aircraft, the cargo area and the passenger cabin (Moreland, 1991; Russell, 1987). Airplane interiors apparently looked like a good resting-place for mosquitoes that bred in the rural, marshy setting of the typical tropical airport (Russell, 1987).

Some of those mosquitoes bit and infected passengers who remained in their seats while their plane was refueling, or they infected passengers in flight or even non-passengers at or near British airports after the plane from the tropics landed. From 1970 to 1985, 23 cases were reported of malaria among people who never even went to a malarious country but were exposed to stowaway mosquitoes (Moreland, 1991 citing White, 1985).

Parasites at Home on Airlines

One British woman barely escaped with her life from an acute case of falciparum malaria that she apparently got from a mosquito bite while traveling from one nonmalarious country to another. The 37-year-old passenger was flying from Johannesburg, South Africa, to Europe in July 1989. While her flight refueled in Abidjan, Cote d'Ivoire, (otherwise known as the Ivory Coast) in West Africa, she stayed in her seat but noticed that the cabin door remained open. A mosquito with malaria in its carry-on must have noticed the same thing and came on board.

Eleven days later, the woman became gravely ill with symptoms of malaria that initially were misdiagnosed as hepatitis. By the time a blood test finally revealed that she indeed was suffering from falciparum malaria, the parasites had invaded 12 percent of her red blood cells. She had cerebral malaria, leading to convulsions and other life threatening complications. She was given exchange transfusions of eight units of blood and other emergency treatment. She recovered, but had to endure a long and difficult convalescence (Oswald, 1990).

In 1983, two passengers boarded an Ethiopian Airliner jet at London's Heathrow Airport for a flight to Rome. Before they got off they were infected with malaria from a stowaway mosquito that must have boarded in Africa (Moreland, 1991).

In the same year, stowaway mosquitoes in or around Gatwick Airport apparently bit two non-travelers and infected them with *P. falciparum.* One of the victims had gone to the airport to visit her husband, who worked there. The other victim only got as close to the airport as a tavern where he was the landlord. The tavern was 10 kilometers, or about 6 miles, west of the airport. The unlucky man suffered critical complications of cerebral malaria, but recovered *(Ibid.)*. Some people thought that mosquito must have taken a car. Maybe a taxi.

Reports Grow for Airplane Malaria

There was even one report of a mosquito riding in a suitcase. The victim was a 67-year-old woman living in Asti in northern Italy, not far from international airports. She had never even been outside her own country. When she became ill, her grave symptoms were similar to other severe infections in nonimmune patients with falciparum malaria. She survived after emergency treatment with blood transfusions, intravenous quinine, chloroquine and corticosteroids. Ten days later she was well.

Doctors were puzzled about a possible mode of transmission in that case. They finally concluded that the mosquito that bit her must have ridden in her daughter-in-law's suitcase. The patient had visited the younger woman when she returned from a trip to Senegal 20 days previously. While abroad, the daughter-in-law had gotten malaria (Rizzo, 1989).

Another mosquito came in on a flight from Africa, got off in London and then boarded a flight to continental Europe, infecting a passenger enroute (Bradley, 1989).

Camp Fire Girls and Korean Malaria

A large category of U.S. travelers didn't have much choice about where they went or what medicines they took to keep well. Those were members of the armed services. Military personnel suffered more malaria than any other group of Americans. Historians figured that throughout U.S. history, more troops were lost to malaria than were lost in combat (Ognibene, 1982).

Even on "peacekeeping" missions, such as the U.S .operation in Somalia in the early 1990s, some personnel had to be evacuated to military hospitals for treatment of malaria (Bartzen, 1993).

Malaria brought to the United States from war or peacekeeping zones only very rarely spread to local populations at home. When it did, the entire U.S. public health system was jolted into action.

One memorable malaria outbreak in California was attributed to parasites from Korea. During the Korean War (June 1950–July 1953), US military doctors became acquainted with "hibernating" malaria parasites. Victims of malaria from temperate or tropical climate zones were struck by those familiar symptoms of fever, chills and pain about two weeks after being bitten by infected mosquitoes. But in Korea, the time between the bite and the symptoms was much much longer, maybe longer than a year (Langmuir, 1963).

Army doctors speculated first that the latency they saw among malaria infections in the troops was due to the human host. That is, maybe the infected men had partial immunity against malaria. Or perhaps they took a preventive drug that had disrupted the parasites' timetable. Whatever the cause, the military doctors added a new preventive or prophylactic drug to the troops' diet that seemed to work against the hibernating strains of the disease. A thorough follow-up on all cases was difficult, however, during the chaos of war.

During a malaria epidemic in the tranquility of a lakeside vacation spot in California, the mystery of Korea's hibernating malaria was observed in detail.[3] The outbreak began at a camp for Camp Fire Girls by the shores of the 15-acre Lake Vera in the foothills of the Sierra Nevada mountains. In early August 1952, three girls living in three separate locations in California came down with vivax malaria (Brunetti, 1954). Their doctors notified public health authorities, who realized at once that they were on the threshold of the first home-based epidemic of malaria since World War II. Notifications then were sent to all doctors throughout the region. Soon the number of malaria victims was up to eight, all widely separated geographically. A ninth victim became sick later in the fall.

Vivax malaria was not as dangerous as falciparum malaria. It was seldom fatal, in spite of the fact that some of the sufferers had episodes of temperature as high as 106 degrees Fahrenheit and violent chills. The urgent problems for the public health sleuths were to figure out how and where the girls got infected and to stop further transmission.

Malaria Goes to Camp

In some ways, the answers were predictable. In some ways, they couldn't have been more bizarre. From the doctors tending the victims, the public health investigators learned the precise dates when each of the girls and young women began suffering symptoms. Those dates were all clustered within a period of days. Doctors knew as well that the onset of symptoms of vivax malaria usually appeared about 12 to 14 days after the bite of an infected mosquito. That meant all the girls would have been infected between about July 15 and 27.

Authorities also discovered early in their investigation that each of the victims had spent part of her summer at the Lake Vera camp, where everyone slept outside on a cot or bedroll. About 1,500 girls and young women between nine and 19 years old stayed at the camp for at least one week each summer. Several staff members stayed on the site, and about 100 people occupied the permanent homes or vacation houses widely spaced along the shores. The mosquito population was abundant, including anophelines that carried the malaria parasite. During the spring and summer there never seemed to be a shortage of mosquitoes near shallow, shaded water.

An urgent question was: were those nine malaria victims actually sleeping by the lake during the critical period in July? Camp administrators confirmed that each camper was there at least part of the period, enough evidence to establish the scene of the crime.

The next urgent question was: how did the mosquitoes get infected? That is, who was the "index person," the person carrying the malaria parasites in his or her blood? That would be the person the mosquitoes fed on before they bit the girls. Health professionals, aware of the typical two-week incubation, returned to the calendar. Counting the days backwards, doctors figured the mosquitoes that infected the Camp Fire girls around the third week of July probably bit a malaria carrier on the shores of Lake Vera around the first ten days of the month. For the sake of the health of the entire community, that carrier had to be identified.

Health workers decided first to check the whereabouts of returned veterans of the Korean War. Several hundred cases of malaria had been reported in California among servicemen home from Korea. The vacation community around the lake was small, so it was not too difficult to find the ex-serviceman whose long 4th of July weekend at the lake had been ruined by an acute relapse of malaria. He had suffered the disease in Korea early in the war, before military doctors had developed their protective protocol for the hibernating strains. In spite of his misery, the veteran stayed as planned at the lake through the holiday weekend.

That was not the end of the story. The public health teams suspected that other people could have been bitten during the third week or so of July and could be turning up at doctors' offices the following spring with fevers, chills and pain.

Health practitioners and authorities were alerted for a possible new wave of victims. Everyone was prepared, but not prepared to see so many infected persons added to the list. A total of 26 latent cases appeared in the spring and summer of 1953, compared with nine victims seen the year before. In addition, six of the nine victims seen the previous year suffered relapses in the summer of 1953. The total number of victims was 35, all from one young man carrying hibernating parasites from Korean malaria in his blood.

Doctors learned several things from the Lake Vera story. They learned that the latency and the relapsing characteristic of the Korean malaria were not due to any partial immunity or prophylaxis in the victims. All had lived their lives in a malaria-free environment. They had no acquired immunity to stall development of parasites they carried. The solution to the mystery was within the parasite itself.

It appeared that the distinctive traits of the Korean parasites had more to do with genetics, a gift from nature to help them survive and produce progeny of their own in spite of the long cruel winters. Parasites produced in the late summer would have a better chance of creating successive generations of young if they arrested their development and spent the winter hibernating in the warm safety of the human host.

In the following spring, they wake up and resume doing what came naturally, perpetuating their species. Those newborn parasites would have enough warm weather ahead of them to thrive and fulfill their obligation to reproduce. There would be enough mosquitoes to deliver the parasites to new hosts, and enough standing water for the newly mature mosquitoes to breed in.

Another lesson from Lake Vera was, never underestimate the tricks of the malaria parasite!

"Cure with Fire" and Other Encounters

The Lake Vera epidemic was followed by a long respite from malaria on the U.S. front. The disease continued to be a frustration for the U.S. military establishment — it always would be — but it dropped out of sight for 20 years or so as a public health problem in the United States.

With the worldwide upswing of the disease starting in 1976, a larger and larger number of Americans in addition to military personnel and tourists were learning first hand about the tropical disease. They included business people, diplomats, missionaries, students, development consultants, Peace Corps volunteers and more. But the numbers of cases remained small.

The largest nonmilitary, susceptible group was people born in malarious regions who entered the U.S. as laborers, or their offspring. They prospered, became U.S. citizens, and later returned to their homelands for a visit. Many former farm laborers from the Punjab in India, for example, became owners of their own commercial farms in the U.S. (Roberto, 1993). Typically, those foreign-born U.S. citizens in California were unaware of the magnitude of the threat of malaria back home. They assumed that the immunity they had acquired years ago was still intact. But they were wrong. Or they believed DDT spraying had permanently controlled malaria back home. Wrong again. Many of those people returned to their new homes in the U.S. with infections of malaria, both falciparum and vivax.

Contaminated Needles

In addition, some people in the U.S. were infected with malaria during blood transfusions. Infections also were reported among the expanding numbers of drug abusers who shared hypodermic needles.

Another kind of high-risk illegal activity was also associated with malaria. Several people with Lyme disease purchased blood infected with *P. vivax* parasites from one of the black markets offering contraband materials with alleged medicinal value. The sick persons deliberately injected the contaminated blood into their veins in the belief that the extremely high fevers of *vivax* malaria would destroy the bacteria responsible for Lyme disease. Afterwards, the sick person presumably would be able to cure the malaria infection with medicines that were still effective.

Before the discovery of antibiotics, that kind of "cure with fire" or "malariotherapy" helped people suffering from advanced stages of syphilis.[4] Both Lyme disease and syphilis were caused by the spirochete group of organisms. The unusual treatment reportedly was successful against syphilis, but results against Lyme disease were inconsistent (USCDC, 1990 & 1991).

Migrant Malaria

Malaria was obviously no stranger in California. Its southern border was a wide open door. Seasonal agricultural workers from Mexico provided the transportation. The workers brought their malaria with them and took it back home across the border at the end of the season.

Many hundreds of poor migrant workers spent the months of May to October working on irrigated farms or construction sites in and around San Diego County across the Tijuana River from Mexico. Typically, they followed the work, moving from site to site as needs arose, living in one flimsy shelter after another.

Most were illegal immigrants, living as "squatters" in secluded clusters beside the streams and estuaries flowing westward to the Pacific Ocean. They worked in the orchards, farms and nurseries that were irrigated by those waters. Some of the workers lived in the open air. Some had shelters they made from cardboard boxes and other discarded materials. Some lived in caves dug out of the hillsides. Practically none of them had access to plumbing.

A large number of the illegal workers were cautious, even secretive. They were victims of several dangerous diseases besides malaria, and their presence made their neighbors — the permanent tax-paying residents — feel uneasy. Some of the residents periodically tried to get the migrants' shelters removed. At the same time, some community leaders tried to pressure the local government or farm owners to provide safe housing for the migrants.

But the system prevailed. Legal American residents were getting a steady supply of fruits and vegetables to eat or export. The workers were well paid, by Mexican standards, and sent most of their earnings to their wives and children back home.

By the 1980s imported malaria was invading glistening luxury neighborhoods among the sunny chaparral hills near the commercial farms. San Diego County Public Health authorities had been aware of the health risks, and they were aware as well that malaria had been rising threefold for four years in Mexico, just across the Tijuana River (Maldonado, 1990; Ginsberg, 1993). But virtually no disease could be monitored nor controlled on a regular basis among such a shifting, elusive population (Ginsberg, 1993; Roberto, 1993). In 1985, 20 cases of malaria were reported to the San Diego County Department of Health Services, but none of the cases aroused suspicion that transmission was occurring on the U.S. side of the border, spreading the disease to others (Maldonado, 1990). Those cases were not linked in clusters of two or more at the same place at the same time. Consequently, health authorities did not fear an epidemic was looming. That is, not until July of 1986.

More Cases From California

The new bad news came from the laboratory at Tri City Hospital in Vista, California, a small city in an area of orchards and farms in northern San Diego County. Five migrant workers had arrived at the hospital on July 4, all acutely ill with vivax malaria. They were suffering from pain and those extraordinarily high fevers. The hospital staff treated them and then let them go (Hunt, 1993; Ginsberg, 1993).

Because of the Independence Day holiday the official health alert was late reaching offices at the San Diego County Department of Health Services. Health authorities were alarmed, realizing at once that such a cluster of infections meant they had an entirely new problem. They had to mount their first ever emergency response to on-going transmission of malaria among people with no fixed addresses. Health authorities knew how fast an epidemic could ignite. They remembered that at Lake Vera just one sick veteran had been responsible for the spread of the disease to at least 35 individuals.

Malaria immediately became the number one priority disease for the rest of the summer and well into the fall. The health workers soon learned that their fears were justified. That cluster of five sick men was indeed just the beginning. Vivax malaria by itself was not life threatening, but if left untreated it might cause grave complications like dehydration, high fever and acute anemia with a low platelet count. Platelets were substances in the blood that allowed it to clot. Persons with a platelet deficit might suffer hemorrhages if they were bruised in a fall.

The health workers assumed the five men were very sick, or else they would not have risked going to a large public facility where authorities might ask to see their immigration papers. Now those original five sick people had to be found, if at all possible. The health team was grateful that at least the group had told the hospital where they worked — at a large array of commercial vegetable farms south of the hospital, near the town of Carlsbad north of the city of San Diego.

The men were among 300 to 400 migrants who tended three farms along the Agua Hedionda Lagoon, a beautiful waterway with lush vegetation and tropical birds. The lagoon, which extended inland from the Pacific Ocean for about two miles, was one of seven estuaries fed by seasonal waters or runoffs from impoundments in the hills.

Workers at each farm were camped along the waters' edges, a site that became a staging area for health authorities stalking the disease. The health team hoped to find the campsites of the five sick men before the mosquitoes did. It wasn't easy locating shelters that were put up with privacy and secrecy in mind, out of view from the roads that wound around the hills and gullies. Authorities couldn't see the encampment until they were about 10 feet away (Mizrahi, 1993). The settlement of 98 migrant workers was on a hillside south of the lagoon, overlooking a tomato farm. One man had dug out a cave for his home. Others had assembled shelters of various pieces of discarded materials, including cardboard, linoleum and blue tarpaulin.

Health Team Was Late

A senior state health official who had investigated malaria outbreaks for 17 years joined the team. He said he had no idea that such a large group of men were living in such bad conditions (Roberto, 1993).

The health team was too late. The original five sick men had moved on, and they were never found. The health workers set up a clinic in a two-door trailer brought in by the farm supervisor. The team was anxious to start checking the remaining migrants before they too scattered. But the team was cautious and sensitive to the fact that the men might be apprehensive about the intrusion. "Everybody was treated well," remembered one of the county nurses. "Nobody acted as if they felt threatened. We just told them we were there for only one reason. That was our genuine concern for their health" (Hunt, 1993). The workers lined up at one door of the trailer. Inside they had their blood drawn, the results to come later. They were interviewed about their recent whereabouts and about other persons not present who might have been sick. They all got chloroquine, which still could prevent or cure vivax malaria, the only malaria species in that region. Then, at the exit door, each got a glass of water to wash down the medicine and a cookie.

Meanwhile, entomologists on the health team set up light traps for mosquitoes along the nearby banks of the lagoon. The scientists discovered several breeding sites of larvae of an unusual mosquito. Back in their labs, the entomologists realized they had discovered a new species of *Anopheles* mosquito, which the team named *Anopheles hermsi.*[5] The new species displayed distinctive characteristics. It preferred the shade of willow trees, and it started looking for human blood each evening about one hour earlier than did the other local mosquitoes (Mizrahi, 1993).

The health team believed that some of the mosquitoes that bred at the water's edge could still have been incubating malaria parasites from blood taken from infected migrants. The specialists applied a larvicide to destroy the larvae, and in the evening the area was "fogged," an insect abatement process that spread a cloud of insecticide over the land. The materials used were derivatives of pyrethrum, a product considered safe around human beings and other animals. Pyrethrum, one of the first insecticides ever used against mosquitoes, was abandoned during the DDT era. It became popular again after use of DDT was banned in the U.S.

Another technique was tried. The control team dug a ditch around a stagnant swampy place among the willows that seemed to be a prime location for mosquito breeding. The new channel drained water from the breeding area, which subsequently dried up. Weed clearance and water diversion projects, although effective in keeping mosquitoes from breeding close to human habitation, reportedly were not popular with real estate and development interests in the area. Permanent residents valued their picturesque environment of wild plant life and migrating birds, and they resisted introduction of unnatural intrusion on the scene *(Ibid.)*.

In other regions and in other times, similar marshes and swamps might have been completely cleared and altered for mosquito control. It made sense for many reasons. Malaria was not the only life-threatening disease that thrived in warm marshes near very poor communities.

Nearby farm managers and permanent residents were notified about the outbreak; they were advised to be on the lookout for sick people and to seek medical help if they themselves came down with symptoms. The health team also let local people know the timetable for the fogging operations, so they could close their houses and stay off the streets if they wanted to.

Tracking the Disease

All of the malaria control activities in the Carlsbad region continued well into the fall, as new victims were found. Besides the visiting state health officials, a team came from the Atlanta headquarters of the U.S. Centers for Disease Control and Prevention to help the local staff.[6] Throughout the period, blood was examined from 321 migrant workers, including workers at the other farms around the lagoon. The health team found a total of 17 new malaria cases and identified nine other cases based on information from hospital records and from interviews with friends and families of victims. Those nine, which included the first five, were never located. All of those 26 infected migrant workers had been residents of the first camp visited. In other words, of the community of 98 people sleeping in that secluded confined area, close to one out of every four was infected in the course of the summer. In addition, two permanent residents of the area had come down with the disease, bringing the total to 28.

The blood smears — many of them sent to Atlanta for detailed analysis — and the interviews convinced the health team that all of the 28 people were infected on the San Diego side of the border, except possibly one of the two permanent residents who had had a recent vacation in Mexico. At least two generations of transmission were involved from June 18 to September 21, making it the first ongoing epidemic of malaria in the U.S. since World War II, as well as the largest outbreak of the disease in the US since the Lake Vera case (Maldonado, 1990).

There were several differences between the two malaria epidemics. At Lake Vera, transmission stopped with just one generation of parasites, the parasites that came from the exserviceman's blood. The victims, even those with the delayed or relapsing onset of symptoms, were easy to find. The episode was easy to contain. The migrants in Carlsbad, in contrast, had no fixed addresses and continued to live in the open near where mosquitoes bred. Transmission lasted throughout the summer.

When the cool fall breezes came to southern California marking an end of the 1986 malaria season, the county health staff was determined to do everything possible to make certain they never again let people with active contagious cases of malaria slip away. A detailed strategy was planned for any future outbreaks. During the summer months the county health staff would periodically notify all health facilities in the area to be on the alert for any new cases. The confirmed cases, or any cases of undiagnosed fever, were to be reported immediately to the health officials.

"We asked them to telephone us immediately — any time, seven days a week, day or night," said Michele Ginsberg, Chief of AIDS and Epidemiology for the county. Ginsberg was especially firm about one point. Health providers were asked not to release any migrant worker who tested positive for malaria until a county health worker had arrived to take him back to his camp. Then the health authorities could monitor his treatment and also could learn immediately and exactly where the disease was being transmitted (Ginsberg, 1993).

The next outbreak in San Diego County came two years later. It was bigger than in 1986, but the entire health community was better prepared. The disease was easier to contain. On August 2, 1988, a migrant worker showed up at a doctor's office in Encinitas, north of the city of San Diego. He was very sick with those agonizing symptoms. His blood smear confirmed he had malaria. He told the doctor that other very sick people were camped near him. The clinician phoned the public health office with the news, then asked the patient to wait for the health authorities. One of the health team said, "We knew if we lost him we would never be able to find the area" (Mizrahi, 1993).

The sick man made his home in the open, under the lemon trees at a canyon encampment about 25 miles north of the city of San Diego. The site was hidden from view of the nearby luxury houses spread across the hills, wide red-tiled roofs radiant in the California sunshine. The familiar makeshift shelters were just five feet from standing water from a small diversion the migrants had created from the nearby stream (USCDC, 1990). Two hours after that call from the local clinic, the health workers were on the scene examining the settlement and interviewing residents. Of the 39 inhabitants, only eight were at the camp. The rest were at their job at a construction site. The health team established that the probable index person for the outbreak was a migrant worker who had camped there several nights in June, had become sick with malaria, and then had left for places unknown.

At dawn the next day, the health workers were back to interview the additional migrants before the truck came to take them to work. Twelve individuals who had the unmistakable symptoms of acute malaria were taken immediately to the hospital. The health team stayed at the hospital with the men, one of whom was particularly ill. The vector control officer was seeing fulminate malaria for the first time. The sick worker was "silent and pale," he said. "Then these intense chills seemed to creep over his whole body until he was shaking violently" (Ibid.). All men in the group tested positive for vivax malaria and were treated. Back at the canyon, the team from the county health office found six more men with malaria and treated them, then gave prophylactic chloroquine to the others. The vector control staff treated the nearby water for larvae.

The team also inspected a camp of migrant workers who lived at a farm on the other side of the road. Seven of them had malaria, as did two additional migrants who worked nearby. The toll was growing to include 19 from the canyon, seven from the farm, and two migrants who lived nearby. Also, two permanent residents of the area acquired the disease. The final total of that outbreak rose to 30 persons, larger than the 1986 epidemic but a lot easier to contain.

The two permanent residents were a surprise. They were a married couple who had just moved from Texas to their new luxury house on a cliff overlooking the canyon. The man was back in Texas on business when he telephoned his wife saying he was sick with fever, aches and chills. Then she came down with the same symptoms and went to the hospital. A blood smear was done immediately. When the presence of malaria parasites was recognized, the doctor called Ginsberg at her home. The attending doctor made the call even before she notified the patient of the findings. It was 10:30 on a Saturday night. Ginsberg recalled she was truly gratified to have more proof that her guidelines were working.

Disease Chooses Luxury Homes

The following year, in 1989, malaria struck again, twice at locations about six miles apart in one of the most luxurious areas in all of San Diego County. First, a 52-year-old banker in a new development at the town of Rancho Santa Fe got sick on July 28. He lived at Fairbanks Ranch in the hills north of the city, a so-called gated community designed to keep everybody who lived there isolated and protected from the outside. Visitors were checked at the security station at the gate where only invited guests, residents, servants and maintenance staff were allowed through.

Inside the gates, beside the large houses of the residents, were outdoor recreation facilities, including a private golf course complete with water hazards. The banker was treated for his malaria, and he recovered without complications. Health workers first did not know where the mosquito that infected him could have come from.

Thirteen days later a migrant from Mexico who worked as a gardener in the banker's community collapsed on the grounds. He was carried to the security station at the gate and then taken to the hospital. He, too, was diagnosed with malaria and treated. Then health workers took the gardener to the riverside encampment where he lived, about one mile from Fairbanks Ranch. Forty other migrant workers in the camp were tested and three were found to be positive for malaria.

Later that summer another man from Rancho Santa Fe got malaria. He was a 32-year-old engineer living in a luxury community six miles northwest of where the banker lived. Health workers trapped *Anopheles hermsi* within a mile of his house and linked the engineer's malaria to the earlier cases of two migrant workers who had camped within a mile of that man's house. But the migrants had already left, for unknown destinations.

In spite of disparity of their economic and social status, the migrant workers and the wealthy residents of San Diego County actually had a lot in common. Both groups lived close to water where malaria vectors bred. Both spent at least part of their evenings outside. The migrants were outside because they had no choice. The more prosperous residents were outside on their patios, or strolling around the scenic hills, or playing golf or tennis. That's why some people moved to those hills in the first place.

Then came a lull. The subsequent three summers passed without any reports of local transmission of malaria. Nothing much had changed to control the disease. Malaria vectors were still breeding along the picturesque waterways. Migrant workers were still living in the open or in flimsy structures with no plumbing.

Farm owners were still not required by law to provide safe

housing for their workers. Malaria was still spreading just across the border in Mexico. Permanent residents were still enjoying their outdoor evening recreation and at least some of them were still trying to get the migrant workers evicted from their neighborhoods. The big difference, and maybe the only difference, might have been the heightened awareness among health providers and among the migrant workers themselves about the constant threat of malaria.

Another positive factor was the new system of good communications between the two groups. In the fall of 1993, county health authorities visited camps of migrants, chatting informally in Spanish, reminding the migrants that the health workers were personally interested in the migrants' well being. The visitors inquired about the migrants' families back in Mexico, and handed out leaflets in Spanish about the symptoms of malaria and about the locations of various health facilities in the region.

One of the oldest and perhaps biggest encampments of Mexican workers in the region, where wives and children lived with the workers, was nestled out of sight between the hills near a large nursery where some of the migrants worked. A school bus was parked on the other side of the small stream that ran by the settlement. Soccer goals were laid out on either side of a bare patch among the shacks. The residences were more substantial and conducive to good health than the cardboard and plastic shelters at other migrant encampments. Many of the residents had planted gardens at their shacks, flowers in front and vegetables in back. There was even a small outdoor restaurant. It was typical of any community in the developing world.[7] Later, a wedding was held there, with a priest officiating. Signs of stability pleased the health workers. At least they knew where the people were. But soon the tranquility was shattered when a demolition team was ordered in to tear down one of the shacks, and new doubts were cast about the future of the settlement. Ginsberg was asked if she thought the personal attention her office was giving to the malaria problem earlier would account for the apparent interruption in disease transmission.

She said, "No. We have just been lucky. Another outbreak could come any time." She also was asked if the county health department had any influence on political leaders to require healthy housing for all people or to alter some of the scenic waterways to make them less hospitable to mosquitoes. She said no, all the health department could do was address health needs and write reports.

It was taken for granted that in San Diego County, as well as in any other community within the United States, episodes of malaria transmission would continue to be rare and not too hard to contain.

It wasn't always that way. In the old days in the United States, malaria was practically everywhere (Duffy, 1992).

---

[1] Malaria was caused by the *Plasmodium* genus of protozoa. The four species of that genus were *P. falciparum, P. vivax, P. malariae,* and *P. ovale.*

[2] See chapter 5, 'The lifestyle of the parasite,' for details about the science of the parasite.

[3] "Epidemic" means a group of infections introduced into a community from the outside. It usually erupts suddenly and with virulence. "Endemic" describes persistent transmission of a disease within the same community. Typically, the endemic disease may be chronic and stable. "Pandemic" means an epidemic of unusual extent and severity.

[4] In 1927, J. Wagner-Jauregg was awarded the Nobel Prize in Medicine for his work treating syphilis with malaria (Desowitz, 1999).

[5] The species was named for William Brodbeck Herms, a scientist who in the early 1900s helped redesign irrigation systems for preventing the breeding of mosquitoes close to human habitat.

[6] Formerly U.S. Centers for Disease Control.

[7] Author's visit. 27 Sep. 1993

Chapter 2
A Land of Opportunity

MALARIA WAS a tropical disease, at home with monsoons, palm trees and year-round sweltering heat. But the disease was versatile. It could strike anywhere if certain conditions were met.

A very specific combination of conditions allowed malaria to sweep into the North American continent, where it made its home for about 240 years. For about 100 of those years, almost the entire span of the continental U.S. was plagued by the disease.

Malaria determined which locations the immigrants chose for their new towns and which places they bypassed. Malaria contributed to the underdevelopment of the South from colonial times until the end of the 1930s, and it probably had something to do with the legendary stoic life style of the early settlers of the nation's Midwest. They had to tame the marshy wilderness while a large share of them were at least a little sick about half the time.

The continents of the New World apparently were free of malaria before the arrival of the Europeans and Africans. Historians believed the earliest known human beings to come to the New World were bands from Asia who followed temporary land routes joining the eastern and western hemispheres during glacial movements dating 15,000 to 20,000 years ago.

Malaria may have parasitized the prehistoric people in Asia by then, but cold conditions on the long migration route would have been a barrier for the malaria parasite, which needed warmth and humidity to complete its entire life cycle, particularly the phase of the cycle that transpired inside a mosquito. Another possible obstacle to the survival of the parasite among the prehistoric migrants may have been the size of their communities; malaria needed large clusters of infected individuals to perpetuate itself. It was believed that those travelers, who became known in the U.S. primarily as the American Indians, moved in small groups (Ortiz de Montellano, 1990). That could explain why American Indians or Native Americans were so very healthy but reportedly nonimmune to many of the common diseases of historic record. Those diseases were brought with invaders from Europe, starting in the late 15th century, or with enslaved Africans who started arriving in the early 16th century (Boyd, 1940; Ortiz de Montellano, 1990).

The New World was a land of opportunity for malaria. Trans-Atlantic ships carried the parasites in the blood of their passengers and crew, and presumably in the bodies of mosquitoes that could survive the voyage. In fact, historians believed many of the ships held enough infected people and mosquito vectors to have full-blown epidemics while still at sea.

The three ships of Christopher Columbus sailed from Palos in a malarious area of southern Spain. They may have carried the disease first to San Salvador in the Bahamas in 1492, and then on to other islands. Columbus wrote frequently about his own fevers. It wasn't long after his arrival that the new Spanish settlements in Santo Domingo were beset by the disease.

In 1510, ships were bringing enslaved Africans to Hispaniola to work in Spain's new overseas sugar industry. The Africans brought their own strains of malaria into the New World (Boyd, 1940). Malaria intensified to such an extent that some historians speculated the disease was responsible for the disappearance of the aboriginal population from the Caribbean islands (Boyd, 1941 citing Childs, 1940).

Soon Spanish and French settlers occupied outposts on the mainland along the southeastern shores of the North American continent, and along the coast of the Gulf of Mexico. It was assumed those people carried malaria in their blood, since it was endemic in many of the regions they came from. But those early settlements of Europeans were small and scattered, and their outposts did not provide the setting malaria needed to thrive.

The picture changed as more immigrants arrived, planted sugar cane and rice along the rich alluvial plains of the Gulf Coast, and imported African slaves to work the plantations.

Colonial Malaria

Among the settlers on the continent, the early colonists from England had the most trouble with malaria. In each new community up and down the Atlantic Coast, tired and undernourished newcomers made their homes from flimsy materials near riverbanks while they cleared forests to put down their first crops. *Anopheles* mosquitoes, the disease's insect vectors, were already ubiquitous. They already had plenty of Native Americans and forest animals to feed on (Boyd, 1941).

In their early letters and reports to home, the settlers from England described the hunger and disease in the New World, frequently mentioning the words "ague," or "intermittent fever," as malaria used to be called.[1]

Malaria may have been brought over on the Mayflower in 1620. Historians could only guess. But big epidemics did strike

31

the Massachusetts colony later, in 1647, 1650, and 1668 (Faust, 1941). By the late seventeenth and early eighteenth centuries malaria was established and thriving all over the New World, and it remained a major cause of sickness and death throughout the colonial period (Duffy, 1992).

Malaria was devastating in the South. The first English settlers sent by Walter Raleigh to colonize Virginia landed in Roanoke in August 1585. There were no reports, however, of illnesses like malaria, presumably because those colonists were mostly recruited from Walter Raleigh's native county of Devon, which was at that time beyond the limits of endemic malaria in England. The story was different when settlers began to arrive from London and from nearby Essex, Surry, Summersetshire and Kent. Malaria was widespread in those places; in fact, another name for malaria was the "Kentish disorder" (Faust, 1945).

The London Company landed in 1607 at Jamestown, and the newcomers tried to make their homes on a small marshy island. A lot of the immigrants weren't up to the challenges of the primitive location in what would become Virginia. One hundred and five colonists were left by the ships on June 22. By the time the ships returned on September 10, forty-six settlers had died. "Ague" was mentioned as the cause of at least one of the deaths. Based on subsequent outbreaks of the disease, historians assumed that just about all of the dead had suffered from malaria (Boyd, 1941).

In 1625, a census was taken in the settlement. Only 1,100 to 1,200 people were left of the estimated 9,000 newcomers. A few hundred had returned to England, but most of the rest died in Virginia from disease or starvation (Duffy, 1979). Eventually, it became apparent that Jamestown was no place to put the capital of the colony of Virginia. The capital was transferred to Williamsburg in 1699 (Boyd, 1941).

A small number of enslaved Africans had begun arriving in Virginia in 1619. By the end of the century, the traffic was heavy. Virginia planters claimed ownership of 200,000 Africans by

1790. During the height of the traffic, from 1680 to 1796, British colonies in America and the West Indies had imported 2,130,000 slaves (Britannica, 1965).

South of Virginia was the new colony of the Carolinas. Nestled in a marshy harbor, its capital Charleston, was like a magnet for malaria. English settlers started to arrive in 1669 and 1670. As the disease swept in, immigration slowed to a trickle. Consequently there simply weren't enough people to sustain a viable colonial capital. Some of the settlers talked about moving the capital to a healthier location. But others, including the management of the new settlement, started a letter-writing campaign to lure more people and enterprises to Charleston. Their correspondence extolled what they described as the extraordinarily healthy climate that awaited new settlers.

One historian, St. Julien Ravenel Childs, researched the period in detail. He said, "If the colony was malarious the settlers possessed amazing skills in concealment, and there was something almost heroic in their deceit" (Childs, 1940).

The malaria spread, but the colony was saved by a new agricultural endeavor, rice. It was a daring choice for such a malarious region. Rice seedlings were imported from Madagascar. Forests were cut to make space for the new venture, and the low lands were inundated. The setting turned out to be exceptional for rice cultivation and also heaven for mosquito larvae. Eventually there was no hiding the fact that the town suffered from full-blown malaria. The news moved up the coast and across the Atlantic.

Many Carolinians gave up, migrating to New York or farther. One Huguenot refugee who immigrated to Boston wrote, "Two young men have just arrived from Carolina [...] they say that they have never seen so miserable a country nor an air so unhealthful. They have fevers all year long from which those attacked seldom recover. If some escape, they become all tawny as are those two who have arrived, who are pitiable to behold..." (*Ibid.*).

The malaria epidemic of 1684 was the worst blow to the Carolinas, taking its highest toll among women and children (Boyd, 1941). Soon immigration was at a standstill, and, ironically, this was fortunate for the colony. An epidemic of malaria could thrive only when stoked by nonimmune individuals. The first infection of a nonimmune typically was the worst. The victim was very sick, and the parasites in his or her blood were most virulent. It usually was the nonimmune newcomer who started a new epidemic in an endemic area. Even if the newcomer were carrying strains of malaria from his or her home country, those strains might be new and dangerous for the other people in the new community. Likewise, the local strains in the adopted setting might make the newcomer very sick. Travel was bad on the health, both for the traveler and for the persons who stayed at home.

Soon Carolina rice was extremely profitable, and the new prosperity made it easier for the prosperous white people to avoid or endure the lingering remnants of endemic disease. Growers had more money. They could afford to leave the work in the wetlands to their slaves or to long-time overseers who had acquired some immunity to malaria. Many growers built luxurious mansions in healthier sections away from the rice. They could maintain their residences well to prevent pools of water from accumulating on their property. Resorts also were established in the nearby hills where Charleston residents could escape the mosquitoes. Those locations remained popular among people all over the East, long after malaria was a threat (Kovacik, 1978).

Reviewing the early period in the history of malaria in the United States, Childs said the Carolina experience revealed "a surprising feebleness in disease when pitted against man's economic desires" (Childs, 1940).

The rice industry spread north almost to the border of Virginia and south to the border of Florida. Malaria spread with it. On the eve of the Revolutionary War, the disease was highly endemic all along the southern Atlantic and Gulf coasts (Faust, 1945).

The War of Independence

The American Revolutionary War, like almost all wars of the world, spread malaria and made it worse. It could thrive on both sides, and it was versatile in selection of breeding spots. The two common species came from separate places. *P. falciparum* came from Africa and remained common in the South. *P. vivax* came from Europe and made its home in the North. Each species existed in multiple strains, which frequently were identified with specific geographic areas. Every strain of each species had its own genetic characteristics, each with distinct immunological markers.[2]

People regularly acquired at least some immunity, if they had been infected frequently with parasites from their local communities. But if the person moved, he or she would likely be nonimmune to the strains of the new area. That was the way epidemics started, according to malariologist John Duffy. It was especially bad if the folks on the move were living out in the open, like pioneers, modern day migrant workers, or those young men and boys camped close to the battlefield. They were likely to get strains of malaria from areas far from home. If they survived, they took the battlefield strains home with them (Duffy, 1992).[3]

In the Revolutionary War, General George Washington's forces besieging Boston in fall of 1775 and General Gates' forces before the battle of Ticonderoga in the summer of 1776 were both plagued by the disease (*Ibid.*).

In the South, nearly an entire garrison came down with malaria at Ebenezer on the Savannah River in an epidemic that also struck forces at the city of Savannah and at Beaufort to the north. British troops were fortified by a large number of mercenary troops from Germany who were incapacitated by the disease following the razing of Savannah. Then malaria struck at Cheraw, in the Carolinas, affecting nearly everyone at the post. The battle of Portsmouth also was complicated by malaria, as was the battle of Yorktown. It was hard for the commanders to pursue a strategy when so many of the troops were sick and couldn't be at the right place at the right time.

By 1776, Cinchona bark from Peru, the substance that quinine was made from, was being widely used in the South. The Continental Congress ordered 300 pounds of it for the troops in the southern department (Boyd, 1941; Duffy, 1992). British troops were using the bark too. A British army surgeon named Robert Jackson, who served on the forces of Lord Cornwallis, was reported to have used the bark "extensively" to treat intermittent fevers among the British forces in their southern campaigns (Boyd, 1941; Faust, 1941). Jackson reported that among troops who did not use the bark, mostly the Hessian mercenaries, there was more death from fevers (Ackerknecht, 1992).

Other infectious diseases stalked the combatants, including small pox, typhoid, typhus and respiratory ailments. Delaware physician James Tilton, who later became Surgeon General of the Army, said 10 to 20 soldiers died from "camp diseases" for every one soldier killed by enemy forces (Duffy, 1992).

Westward Expansion

After independence, the frontiers of the new nation expanded, sweeping malaria in a multitude of strains from East to West, in and out of almost all corners of the expanding country, leaving no area untouched except the Rocky Mountains and Maine (Boyd, 1941; Faust, 1941; Duffy, 1992). Malaria always was a good traveler.

The depth of the suffering could be seen in the wealth of details from memoirs, letters and articles in medical journals. The extent of the disease would seem almost incredible to the reader.

Malaria went west with the traders, miners and pioneers, passing through Indian territory and frontier Army posts, where outbreaks of the disease were not uncommon. Fort Gibson in Oklahoma was hard hit and became known as the "charnel house of the Army" (Faust, 1941, p. 186).

Newcomers from the South and the East brought new strains of the disease to the Sacramento-San Joaquin valleys in California. Two groups were predominately responsible for those serious outbreaks. Spanish immigrants from Mexico set up new prosperous agricultural enterprises, selling fruit and vegetable produce to dealers all across the country. The farmers also brought with them their own irrigation techniques, creating popular breeding places for malaria vectors.

When big gold strikes lured miners or would-be miners from the East to California, malaria thrived in the new venue. The eastern miners introduced still more strains of the disease, causing new waves of suffering. In many locations miners set up hydraulic methods for separating gold, leaving new pools of standing water near places where the miners slept in makeshift shelters (Boyd, 1941). Some malaria from the inland mining regions reportedly showed up in the city of San Francisco (Roberto, 1993). Finally, malaria became so virulent in two Army posts in California that they had to be abandoned. Those were Camp Far West in 1852, and Camp Reading in 1856 (Herms, 1940).

The disease broke out as well in the Columbia River valley in the Northwest. An epidemic on the lower Columbia in 1829–1832 was a disaster for the Indians. Nine-tenths of the indigenous population died and some tribes were exterminated (Boyd, 1940). In those outer, western reaches of malaria, population clusters were thinly spread, and the disease typically struck and departed quickly.

During that same period, between the Revolutionary War and the Civil War 85 years later, malaria appeared often in the Northeast among people who hadn't taken part in the early westward treks. Some of the most vulnerable areas were new communities in northern Pennsylvania and New York, all along the southern shores of Lakes Huron, Erie and Ontario, and the valleys of the St. Lawrence, Hudson and Mohawk Rivers. Workers digging the Erie Canal suffered badly from the disease, as did the nearby residents. Even neighboring communities in Canada were affected.

Manhattan residents suffered a startling malaria epidemic in the early 1800s. The disease was unleashed when a new grid-iron street pattern was laid out. That pattern blocked the natural drainage of the streets, creating stagnant pools that brought mosquitoes closer to residential communities (Boyd, 1941).

While malaria was erupting and subsiding in isolated locations in the Northeast and the West, different epidemiological patterns were emerging elsewhere. The disease was coalescing, creating two distinct images in the two wide geographic regions where most of the population was sick for at least some of the time. It was becoming apparent that malaria was a local disease, dependent on specific ecological and social conditions for its spread and for its control.

Endemic malaria smoldered in the South from colonial times until about 1940. The climate was congenial to many tropical diseases, and the dangerous falciparum malaria was common. That southern setting was a marked contrast to what became known as "frontier malaria," which came in a series of fiery epidemics following homesteaders into the Midwest. After the Midwest became settled and prosperous, malaria retreated quickly. The same thing happened in the South; it just took longer.

Malaria Among the Homesteaders

Malaria epidemics of the upper Mississippi River Basin of the Midwest were ignited by the huge waves of pioneers from poverty-stricken areas of Europe and from congested, unhealthy eastern cities of the United States where prospects for poor immigrants were not good.

The central and midwestern regions they chose to occupy offered a new set of challenges. The upper Mississippi River Basin, comprising Minnesota, Wisconsin, Iowa, Missouri and Illinois, was sculpted by glaciers that had crept southward thousands of years in the past, creating the Great Lakes and lesser lakes and bowls. The land between the lakes was streaked by rivers and streams emptying into the great Mississippi. What was left for the new farmers were mainly marshy forests and swampy prairies.

The Mississippi River drainage basin covered 1,255,000 square miles, or 3,250,000 square kilometers, the third largest drainage basin in the world after the Amazon Basin and the Niger River Basin. The Mississippi Basin was more erratic than the other two, by far. The origin of its waters was an immense apron of snow-covered mountains and prairies, with a spring run-off that spilled water far beyond the riverbanks. Most of the seasonally flooded areas never had time to dry up completely.

The upper Mississippi Basin was an exotic vision. Its swamps contained lush expanses of wild rice, big animals with thick warm coats, slinky animals with lush silky coats, migratory waterfowl and mosquitoes. Mosquitoes were most abundant in the fall when the seasonal waterways created by spring floods became shallow and still (Boyd, 1941).

Virtually the entire region was the hunting and trading territory for many tribes of Indians. The heart of the region, penetrated by French missionaries, trappers and traders starting in 1673, was the wide Mississippi north of its junction with the Missouri River. Here were the villages and lodges of Indians of the Illinois Confederation. The French people called it Illinois Country.

It was not known if the French brought any malaria with them. If they had, it didn't take hold in the New World setting. Their communities apparently were not so densely populated as to allow sustained transmission of the disease. At least the French settlers didn't mention any serious patterns of disease problems in their letters and journals. They did write passionately, however, about the hardships inflicted by the clouds of voracious mosquitoes. The wet woodlands always were appealing to mosquitoes. One Jesuit priest wrote in 1772 that "the little insect has caused more swearing since the French have been in Mississippi than had previously taken place in all the rest of the world" (Boyd, 1941; Ackerknecht, 1945).

The explorers also reported that the Indians they encountered were just as tormented by the mosquitoes as they were. Father Jacques Marquette wrote about contraptions devised by Indians near the mouth of the Missouri River to protect themselves from the insects (Ackerknecht, 1945).

After Independence, new settlers from eastern U.S. cities and from Europe began to appear, in small groups at first, following eastern rivers to the Allegheny Mountains, then over and down into the Mississippi River Basin. The route continued along the Ohio River until it reached the soggy forests of the Mississippi Basin that were virtually free for the taking. Before long, a truly gigantic migration was underway, the numbers quickly rising to several million. As a group, the pioneers were poor; they came carrying their few belongings on their backs, on their pack animals, or in covered wagons. Many of them carried strains of malaria in their blood, a wide variety of strains of disease organisms from the various European homelands of the settlers and from some of the American locations they were passing through. The settlers, infected and noninfected alike, camped beside the rivers to rest, giving mosquitoes the opportunity to mix up the various strains of the disease and bring on acute suffering.

Many of the settlers were very ill when they reached their new homesteads. Typically, the family's first dwelling was a semi-open shack beside the water. As newcomers cleared their land and their settlements grew, new full-blown epidemics of malaria erupted. It was the same dynamics of transmission as in wartime, with people gathered from many locations, living in flimsy shelters in an unstable environment near where mosquitoes bred.

But one factor was different. At the end of the trip, those people had their own land. It was waterlogged and full of mosquitoes, but it was theirs. They also had realistic expectations that better times lay ahead.

By the early 1800s malaria was scattered throughout the Midwest. Some places suffered more than others, and southern Illinois was one of the worst. The glaciation that carved out the Great Lakes left Illinois pockmarked with shallow bowls that were prime breeding places for mosquitoes.

One early traveler described southern Illinois in the spring, when the swollen rivers flooded the low prairies for miles and miles. Looking across the water one could see wild rice and other aquatic plants reaching over the surface, while canoes carried people to and fro on their routine business *(Ibid.)*. Illinois quickly became notorious even to people back East as being extremely malarious. An early governor, John Reynolds, wrote that from 1800 to 1805 Illinois was known as a graveyard (Levine, 1964). In Pike County, for example, a malaria epidemic killed 80 percent of the early settlers in the 1820s.

Many people decided to stay away, prematurely ending their westward trek. That decision was a boon to one community along the big northern bend of the Ohio River. At that reportedly malaria-free location, many trekkers decided not to go any farther. Their new home became the prosperous city of Cincinnati (Ackerknecht, 1945).

Obviously, a lot of settlers trudged on to Illinois anyway and joined the ranks of the malaria victims. Two doctors in one county treated 1,500 cases of malaria in 1846, and reported that the disease had become even worse during the severe epidemic that followed the unusually wet summer of 1849.

St. Louis, Missouri, also acquired a bad reputation. Many settlers who tried to live there packed up and left. But the allure of the valuable location at the junction of the two great rivers, malarious or not, always drew new settlers in. In fact, figures from that city apparently illustrated the relationship between an influx of settlers and the prevalence of malaria. The year 1852 saw a 30 percent increase from the previous year in the number of new immigrants, with a correspondingly large increase in the disease's prevalence.

Two other sets of numbers helped illuminate the dimensions of the migration. In 1810, Illinois had a population of 12,282. By 1880, the figure was 3,077,871. In Missouri, the 1820 figure was 20,845. The population in 1880 was 2,168,380 *(Ibid.)*. Those waves of immigration were following waves of economic chaos elsewhere. The invasion of settlers reached its crescendo from 1830 to 1860, with one of the biggest influxes following the 1837 financial crisis in Europe. Then, 20 years later, another big boost in new settlers followed the financial panic in the U.S. in 1857 *(Ibid.)*.

The disease kept spreading and gaining power as settlers continued along the thoroughfares of tributary rivers deeper into the midwestern wilderness, setting up new communities, clearing their land and building their log cabins. Many had become at least partially immune to the malaria they brought with them, but they were constantly threatened by the new strains carried by the people who followed them *(Ibid.)*.

That pattern lasted until the migrations stopped. New big public works programs were installed to contain flooding for agricultural development and land was cleared and drained for crops. Then settlers began to earn enough to build solid houses and find ways to distance themselves from places where mosquitoes bred.

Michigan created one of the early programs for making the land more suitable for settlement and agriculture. In 1857, the state adopted legislation to encourage drainage of swamps, marshes and lowlands, a public policy that also worked to evict malaria vectors that bred in the waters (Boyd, 1941). The positive health aspects of that and other drainage projects were attracting wide attention. In 1874, the American Medical Association devoted a meeting to this topic.

Health Care

Just how many people became ill with malaria? The region it covered was very widespread, and within the communities it was very, very common. There were, however, no reliable statistics for the period (Faust, 1941). It would be well into the next century before the Public Health Service was established and authorities started trying to gather data about the prevalence of malaria. Even then, counting all the people in remote rural areas who were sick with malaria was almost as hard as counting the people who had a bad cold.

Nevertheless, letters, journals and reports from doctors and others contained some helpful anecdotes and characterizations, such as "almost everyone was sick" with malaria, and "the whole family suffered every summer" (Ackerknecht, 1945). One historian who painstakingly researched the malaria of the period said, "No part of the Mississippi Valley escaped its ravages" (Faust, 1941).

Many of malaria's victims must have been acutely ill, since so much of the population was periodically encountering what were to them new strains of the disease. However, in a temperate climate such as the Midwest, people could expect relief during the cold winter months. They had a chance to recuperate and become strong again before the next waves of infection struck.

Letters and journals from the period seemed to reveal a kind of stoic acceptance of the disease as part of the price or tax to pay for life on the frontier. They were people who had already endured and witnessed a lot of suffering just to reach their new homes. Many were victims of famine in their home countries and had survived the filth and dangers in the big cities of the East and the arduous overland travels across the country.

Soon, harbingers appeared of better times ahead. For instance, it became apparent that the newly drained farmland of the Midwest was spectacularly good for cereal crops. The states of Ohio, Indiana, Illinois, Wisconsin and Iowa produced one-fourth of the wheat and corn supply in the entire country in 1839, and within 20 years the ratio had risen to one-half. After another 20 years of that kind of economic growth, malaria finally started its retreat.

Malaria Takes the South

Malaria in the post- independent South behaved differently from the frontier malaria of the Midwest and the malaria in other regions of the country where short but violent epidemics were the norm.

The South continued to have its share of epidemics, but most of the malaria there just held a persistent, low, steady posture. After a number of infections, people were able to acquire partial immunity, and endemic, chronic malaria set in. That meant that their immune systems had to keep fighting the disease to maintain stable health.

People who suffered from chronic malaria were particularly vulnerable to other diseases. Their immune systems were less than fully effective against tuberculosis, for instance, or against measles, hookworm and typhoid. Those partially immune people in endemic areas had to fortify their defenses constantly against malaria. Consequently other diseases often were unchallenged. So while malaria seemed to bother many Southerners less and less, they had more than their share of other ailments, and they never had a chance to regain the stamina that was their birthright (Carter, 1919; Najera, 1996).

The endemic low-intensity malaria that lingered in some pockets of rural poverty until about 1940 marked the destiny of Southern life and trapped many people in a vicious cycle. The South was poor because malaria was widespread, and malaria was widespread because the South was poor. Other important factors, of course, influenced the high incidence of malaria in the South. The climate was warm and humid, somewhat akin to

44

the tropical climates where malaria was most at home, and Southerners had to contend with falciparum as well as vivax malaria.

The South was also handicapped by poor soil. Over much of the land the topsoil was quite shallow, in contrast to the rich topsoil of the Midwest that was often many feet deep. Several generations of Southerners engaged in trial - and - error farming before they could create successful agricultural patterns that permitted farming populations to stay in one place and save a little money to invest in their health and future.

All along the middle coast various crops were tried and abandoned, leaving people and their land worn out and unhealthy. During the early 1800s, many coastal people moved inland to newly settled land in the Piedmont region, taking their slaves and their malaria with them. Serious outbreaks of malaria were reported in that region between 1833 and 1837. An economic depression followed, and many people returned to resettle the homesteads they had abandoned. The routes leading back took them through unplowed land, vegetative debris and the pools of stagnant water where mosquitoes chose to breed.

In addition to the migrations between the coast and the Piedmont, many people began moving farther south and west into Kentucky, Tennessee, Alabama, Mississippi, Arkansas and northern Louisiana. Sometimes the farmers sold their enslaved Africans before departing, but other times they took them along, compounding everybody's risk of new malaria outbreaks.

Meanwhile, new French settlers were bringing their own strains of the disease from France to Mobile, New Orleans and Natchez (Faust, 1941). Alabama endured particularly grave problems during the 1820s. Several epidemics struck as more people moved into the state and cleared land for development. Two of Alabama's early capitals had to be abandoned because of malaria (Duffy, 1992).

Rice, cotton and tobacco were the main crops in the old South, and all three demanded a lot from the owners and their slaves. Each of the three crops created different disease hazards.

At first, tobacco cultivation actually helped control the spread of malaria. In Virginia, tobacco thrived in small patches on well-drained land. There was no place for mosquitoes to breed on an immaculately tended tobacco farm. In fact, some people found in later times that the chopped-up tobacco leaves worked as a larvicide to keep mosquitoes from breeding in nearby ponds.

But tobacco wore out the land. Many early tobacco farmers in Virginia failed after a few years, and the owners abandoned their farms. Some of their enslaved Africans were sold to plantation owners in the Louisiana bayou, where malaria subsequently intensified, or to rice producers along the coast. But tobacco eventually brought a lot of money to Virginia and North Carolina after the farmers had acquired a better understanding of the demanding crop and discovered practical ways to drain the farms and keep their homes a good distance from the breeding mosquitoes.

Rice continued to be a very profitable but unhealthy crop in the early days. Growers in coastal cities such as Savannah, Georgia followed the example of Charleston producers by planting in tidal swamps adjacent to the city. And just as had happened in Charleston, malaria in the new locations became a terrible menace. By 1805, malaria-related deaths and chronic illness were so common that the flow of European immigrants to Savannah started to dry up, and the city's prosperity was jeopardized (Cassidy, 1989).

Savannah's City Council decided that it could not risk losing the new immigrant populations the city needed so badly for cheap labor and economic growth. In 1817, local government mandated that swamps near residential areas be drained and cleared, using tax money to complete the project and to compensate rice producers for their losses (Boyd, 1941). But even these desperate measures did not solve the city's malaria problems; medical reports indicated that Savannah during the 1820s and 1830s was a "malarial pocket," with a death rate of 70 per 1,000 people sick with the disease (Cone, 1979).

Cotton was a big moneymaker that was well suited to the South, but it required considerably more slave labor than the other crops discussed here. In boom years, when additional slaves had to be purchased and moved into already crowded shanties, malaria rose throughout the plantations and larger communities.

Doctors in the South became aware that the African workers who were moved from one region to another often required some "seasoning" while they recuperated from infections of malaria in the new region (Warner, 1989). It was apparent that the slaves did not suffer as much in those moves as did the white owners and their families. The reason for this difference, doctors speculated, was that some slaves still had immunity to strains of malaria that they or their ancestors had brought from Africa. In a way, the doctors were right, although scientific corroboration did not come until 1910. Many Africans did have a kind of built-in protection against malaria — namely, the deformed red blood cell called sickle cell that could not be penetrated by the malaria parasite. People with that trait had some protection from malaria, but if they inherited the trait from both parents, they could develop the life-threatening disease called sickle cell anemia.

Disease and Optimism

American doctors, like their colleagues in Europe, treated malaria in two ways, irrationally and rationally. Until the early to mid-1800s, treatments for malaria were the same extreme measures most doctors used against many severe afflictions. Since it was widely believed most internal ailments were caused by internal imbalances in the patient's life forces, draining out the excesses that tipped the balance seemed to make sense. Often patients were given harsh substances to purge their systems by vomiting or vacating the bowels. The most drastic of the irrational treatments was bloodletting. Even the most prominent doctors would routinely lance a patient's artery to drain off some blood when it was determined there was an excess (Warner, 1989).

Several reform - minded doctors, however, were beginning to demand an end to old, seemingly barbaric practices. But since no obvious alternative "cures" for malaria were available, the purging and lancing continued. Some doctors also prescribed medications for malaria, but many of those sounded barbaric to modern ears. They included arsenic potions, opiates and narcotics for pain and "nerves," and calomel salts, a mixture of mercury and chlorine.

Most of malaria's victims were poor, and doctors were few. Consequently the great majority of the population never received professional care for malaria. Maybe they were the lucky ones. Many people treated themselves with popular concoctions sold informally. Some families used homemade medicinal teas prepared from the powdered bark of the slippery elm, sassafras, cinchona and other trees.

Rational treatment for malaria began when quinine was produced by French chemists in 1820 and then manufactured in Philadelphia three years later. It was the first substance in Western medicine that was effective against a specific disease. For the first several years in the U.S., however, results were disappointing. Historians suspected doctors were prescribing inadequate doses of the new drug.

That changed after the U.S. Army's well-publicized experience in Florida in the second Seminole War (1835–1842.) In their assignment to drive Seminole Indians out of their homelands in Florida, many troops suffered critical malaria. They were cured and accomplished their mission after treatments with experimentally large doses of quinine. By the 1850s, the old barbaric practices were abandoned, and the larger doses of quinine were standard treatment (Ackerknecht, 1945).

After the Civil War, during the 1860s, doctors and consumers in the North and the South used huge amounts of quinine with reputed success, and the drug's popularity soared. Historians reported that by the 1870s quinine was on the shelf of every family who could afford it. Almost half of the quinine produced worldwide in 1888 was used in the United States *(Ibid)*.

Many people in malarial parts of the country took a spoonful a day, even when they weren't suffering from any of the classic symptoms. Some enthusiasts routinely cut the bitter taste of quinine by mixing it with their coffee or with alcoholic beverages (Barber, 1929). And some families and individuals combined quinine with other "cures," such as arsenic and calomel. It was not rare to hear of a case of arsenic poisoning during malaria epidemics (Ackerknecht, 1945).

In many places, mainly in the South, quinine and calomel were mixed in a powder. One man remembered the custom from his boyhood in Louisville, Kentucky. He said, "Whenever we seemed at all unwell we received immediately 10 grains of quinine with calomel in powder form on the point of a knife. Some of the older people had lost their teeth from excessive doses of calomel" *(Ibid.)*.

People became passionately loyal to quinine. One survivor of an epidemic in the fall of 1838 in Palmyra, Michigan wrote: "Had our bread failed, our wells and rivers dried up, we could have endured it. But to be without cathartic pills and quinine would be worse than a bread and water famine" *(Ibid.)*.

U.S. Army doctors quickly came to use quinine as a diagnostic test: if the patient didn't get quick relief from the familiar symptoms, then he or she probably didn't have malaria (Boyd, 1941). And quinine remained the first-choice or only remedy in the armed forces for many years, although it eventually became apparent that the medicine did not really cure malaria. It suppressed the parasites and reduced or temporarily eliminated the symptoms. Within a short period, the people who were "cured" were usually sick again. It was learned later that quinine also suppressed the body's capacity to acquire some immunity to the disease. People usually could expect some temporary or partial immunity after a case of malaria, but not if they had been taking quinine. That was why they needed the medicine so often (Nelson, 1941; Russell, 1943; Tigertt, 1972).

Big Market for Quinine

It didn't take long for the makers of patent medicines to exploit quinine. Many of the labels proclaimed a new "secret ingredient," and usually that ingredient was quinine. Since even a small dose of quinine would make the sick person feel at least a little better for a short time, the nostrums were in great demand.

The names of those "medicines" evoked images of horse-drawn buggies, board sidewalks and pickle barrels: Dr. Cyrenius Wakefield's "famous treatment for chills and fever;" Roman's Tonic Mixture; and Ring's Remedy, "guaranteed to cure fever and ague." The most popular was Dr. J. Sappington's "antifever pills." Doctors reflecting on those early days believed that the only real benefit of those remedies was a kind of placebo effect or psychological boost. At least people could feel as if they were "doing something" about malaria. The producers made a lot of money, for the obvious reason that consumers felt they had to take such drugs almost constantly.

Quinine, either in pure form or in various nostrums, was used in the United States right up until the early 1940s. Then the drug became popular again in various areas during the 1970s and 1980s, after other modern synthetic drugs that had replaced quinine lost their efficacy. In that later period, quinine was mainly used in combination with other substances. By the 1990s quinine combinations were being credited for saving lives of many acutely ill patients throughout the world.

Southern Doctors

Any historic survey of malaria in the United States had to examine closely the role of early Southern doctors in the understanding and eventual control of the disease. Southern doctors as a group were intensely curious both about possible clues to explain the functions of malaria and about environmental factors that might have been responsible for outbreaks and epidemics.

Some doctors perpetuated the belief that Southerners were not as robust as northerners. They sought explanations for the differences and ways to compensate for them. For example, bloodletting was not used as often in the South as it was in the North; many doctors believed that Southerners were too frail for that treatment (Warner, 1989). On the other hand, doctors in the South used quinine and calomel in larger doses than did their colleagues in the North; they figured that people in the South were so weakened by malaria, they needed more medicine to gain any benefit.

Southerners had respect for their physicians, but they didn't get to see them often. The physicians were widely scattered over the immense and sprawling farmlands of the South. Typically, the plantation owner's wife supervised the health care for the enslaved Africans. Or one of the enslaved women was trained to nurse others in the slave quarters. For those duties and other home doctoring many people relied on the various manuals that the Southern doctors published. Two important and ubiquitous topics in those documents were malaria and yellow fever, also transmitted by a certain kind of mosquito. The overriding theme was that the average person, if provided with accurate information, could take care of his or her own health (Keeney, 1989).

But the most significant contribution of Southern doctors to the modern understanding of malaria control was their fervid interest in understanding and explaining the environmental peculiarities of the region and its disease patterns. That interest motivated their search for practical ways to alter the environment effectively to evade or control the disease.

The fascination began as early as the middle 1700s. The South, with its semi-tropical flora, fauna and climate, was an exotic place to live for most people from Europe. Many of the doctors made copious notes about weather patterns, vegetation, soil conditions, mineralogy, geological formations and patterns of waterways and of wildlife. They also gathered information about the lifestyle of Indians. Nothing seemed too insignificant to record in the search for new ways to explain the high prevalence of fevers and other common, destructive human conditions that seemed to harm Southerners more than Northerners. That was before people understood the role of germs as disease agents, before high-definition microscopes, and before the science of biochemistry was developed. For the doctors of the South, their environment was their lab.

The quest for environmental links with disease, a quest that was seen to a lesser extent in the North and in Europe, was referred to as "vigorous neo-Hippocratic environmentalism." Hippocrates was the Greek doctor from the fifth century BC who was known as "The Father of Medicine."[4]

Some members of the growing Southern school of medicine in the us pointed out that the island of Cos in the Aegean Sea, where Hippocrates worked, was geographically similar to their own home region. Cos lay between the 36th and 37th latitudes, the same zone occupied in the North American continent by southern Virginia and northern North Carolina (Cassidy, 1989; Warner, 1989).

Pioneer Doctors

One frontier neo-Hippocratic practitioner was Daniel Drake. He was born in 1785 in New Jersey. Three years later he traveled with his family in two horse-drawn wagons across the Alleghenies, then on a boat down the Ohio River and finally on to the area that became Maysville, Kentucky.

When he was nine, his father and he split logs and built their house. Hauling the logs by horse to the homestead gave the young Drake a chance to study his environment. Out in the woods, his father would hoist him up on to the horse. The boy pulled the newly cut log to the house site, rolled off the animal and unhitched the log. Then, since he wasn't big enough to get back on the horse by himself, the boy would walk the horse back into the woods where his father was working. Drake was fascinated by all the peculiarities, similarities, changes and inconsistencies in this natural setting, and he was preoccupied for the next five years with noting, collating and processing details of what he saw. His father realized the boy was precocious, and in 1800 the two walked for two days to Cincinnati. There the father turned his fifteen-year-old son over to a local doctor as an apprentice.

After Drake himself joined the faculty at the medical school in Louisville, Kentucky, he continued his observations in medical geography, teaching in the winter and traveling most of the rest of the time. He covered 30,000 miles over a 10-year period. In 1850, his observations were collected in a unique work he called *A Systematic Treatise, Historical, Etiological and Practical, on the Principal Diseases of the Interior Valley of the North America, as they Appear in the Caucasian, African, Indian and Esquimaus Varieties of its Population.* The passages relating to malaria were preserved in a volume published by the University of Illinois Press in 1964 (Levine, 1964).

Drake called malaria "the great cause of mortality or infirmity," justifying his conclusion with precise observations. What he didn't mention in his book was that his own wife died of malaria (Levine, 1964).

"It is well known," Drake wrote, "that a family may settle down in the forest and cultivating but a small spot remain free from fever; but when several families arrive, and an extensive breaking up of the soil takes place, it [the fever] immediately begins to prevail, although the heat and moisture are thereby not increased" (Levine, 1964, p 717). He thus saw that malaria required warm temperatures and proximity to water. He also made the important discovery that malaria was apparently dependent on the presence of a large number of people to propagate itself.

In addition, Drake became aware that malaria was synchronized with the behavior of the Mississippi and Missouri rivers, especially near their junction at St. Louis. He said that area had more malaria, or "autumnal fever," than any other part of the valley. "We ascend the Mississippi to the mouth of the Missouri," he wrote, "and we find its annual floods leaving small lakes, ponds, swamps and lagoons, which in the aggregate are of great extent and but partially drained or dried up before the next inundation." The partially dried-up pools of water, he concluded, were connected with the dominance of malaria in this region (Levine, 1964.).

Many people in those days still clung to the idea that malaria was caused by a kind of poisonous vapor commonly called "miasma." It was thought that such vapors emanated in the evening from the decomposing organic matter in swamps and pools of standing water. They also believed that the forest had a mediating effect on the vapors, that the leaves of the trees could absorb the toxic vapors and prevent the disease. According to that theory, when settlers cleared trees to build their houses and plant their crops, they were giving the disease a free hand.

But Drake's reasoning was not that simple. He wrote with prescience that, "While water is essential to the production of this fever, other causes must cooperate to give it power." And he believed an "instinctive propensity of the human mind" would ultimately lead humankind to the discovery of a single efficient cause for malaria.

Drake became an early and outspoken advocate among the small group of physicians and naturalists in the South and elsewhere who were building a case against the mosquito, an indictment that was based on observations and common sense long before any scientific explanations were available.

It was reasonable to speculate that the special concerns of Southern doctors as a group had a lot to do with the early signs of improvement in the status of malaria control in the South in the years just preceding the Civil War. And the improvement, although temporary, was indeed real. Conditions in the South had begun to stabilize; communities were staying put; viable farming methods had taken hold; and many people were acquiring enough resources to keep their land tilled and drained. It was believed that malaria was finally beginning to relax its hot grip on the South.

The small improvements were wiped out by the devastating "War Between the States." The shadow of the Southern neo-Hippocrates movement could be recognized later, however, after the war, when doctors from the South assumed a creative and profound role in finding practical ways to eliminate old pockets of endemic malaria in remote, poor, rural regions through public health projects. It was those projects in the South, plus the prosperity that eventually followed, that finally drove malaria away for good (Boyd, 1941).

The Civil War

The American Civil War of 1861 to 1865 revitalized malaria. The total number of malaria cases suffered by white troops in the Northern armies were reported to be 1,163,814. Reports said 8,140 of those troops died of the disease (Ognibene, 1982 citing Charles Smart, 1888). The casualty reports, however, were suspect. In communities with endemic malaria, it was common that troops came from all directions, bringing with them an assortment of local strains of the disease. Troops from both sides camped in the open on the outskirts of battlefields, allowing mosquitoes to infect them with strains for which the troops were nonimmune.

Malaria was endemic in much of the region occupied by war. Typically, men and boys who survived the disease then carried the new strains back to their home territories, causing new epidemics of virulent disease to erupt across the map.

War allowed army doctors to see in raw clarity the disease that in peacetime was usually out of sight, hidden in remote communities of the rural poor, or in slave quarters, or at the riverside camps. Army doctors reportedly saw troops shaking so hard with malaria they couldn't stand up, and they saw young men die of malaria by the thousands.

Until the twentieth century, few statistics were collected for analyzing the patterns of the disease in times of peace. In times of war, the casualties were counted.

Wars put malaria on the scorecards. But for the Civil War there was only one scorecard, the record of diseases and deaths among the Northern forces

One of the worst battle zone epidemics was at a Confederate river battery below Savannah, Georgia. That epidemic lasted from October 1862 to December 1863, and was responsible for some seemingly illogical statistics. One unit of 878 officers and men endured 3,313 cases of malaria during the 15-month period (Boyd, 1941 citing Charles Smart, 1888).

Observers pointed out that many of the victims kept getting reinfected or suffered recurrences from the same persistent infections. The high figures included replacements for men who left their units because of malaria. The replacements were then new targets for the disease. Since the Northern army was consuming great quantities of quinine, it was obvious that the drug was not being well administered or that the parasite had already developed tolerance to the drug, or both. Doctors were realizing that a quinine "cure" for malaria did not protect the victim from future infections.

Malaria statistics were usually unreliable, according to one malariologist of the early 20th century, Ernest C. Faust of the Tulane University. He summed up the reasons at a symposium on human malaria in 1941. He cited the poor records of malaria spleen surveys; the inability of many doctors to recognize malaria in a sick population; the common practice of self-diagnosis and self-treatment; and the prescription of antimalarials without adequate diagnosis.

The post-war period was extremely difficult for Southern civilians. It took the South about 75 years to recover economically. But economic recovery, along with other factors, finally led to relief from malaria throughout the region.

---

[1] Early settlers also suffered from typhoid, typhus, cholera, yellow fever and starvation. Historians had several reasons for assuming that malaria was by far the most common disease: the familiar episodic rhythm of the high fever and violent chills, the association with the malaria back home, and the subsequent patterns of its dispersal in the new locations.

[2] A strain is defined as a selected group of organisms sharing or presumed to share a common ancestry and usually lacking clear-cut morphological distinctions from related forms but having distinguishing physiological qualities (*Webster's Third New International Dictionary, 1963*).

[3] Many scientists believed that the story of strains wasn't as simple as it seemed. There was disagreement among scientists about immunity to different strains. Some said that immunity was not strain-specific and immunity to one strain of *P. falciparum* would make the individual immune to other strains of *P. falciparum*. Others sited examples from various U.S. locations contradicting the above assumption and said that it was conceivable that isolated populations of parasite in certain locations were different enough to cause illness in immune people. As one scientist put it on the malaria discussion group of the 'WHO malaria database' web-site, "Our field, malaria, is full of conflicting and contradictory reports."

[4] See chapter 6, for more on Hippocrates.

Chapter 3
Creeping Prosperity

I N 1865, when the guns were silenced and dust had settled on the Civil War battlefields, malaria was still around. Three distinct geographic patterns of the disease prevailed.

In the West, malaria was no longer a public health threat except for California's limited and controllable outbreaks among the vast irrigated farms.

In the northeastern states, some returning veterans brought their malaria home with them, setting off a few limited outbreaks. Southern strains of virulent *P. falciparum* could not sustain transmission long in the temperate climate up North. Occasionally a new public works project disrupted the landscape, temporarily allowing mosquitoes to breed close to residential areas and spread the disease. Those new fires were quickly contained.

In the upper Mississippi River Basin, signs of new prosperity were everywhere, even in Illinois. Most of the tillable land had been occupied and tilled. The influx of new settlers, carrying strains of malaria from far-flung places, had slowed. Many farmers earned enough money to build sturdy houses away from the riverbanks. In that vast area once so heavily infected, independence from malaria was not so wild a dream (Boyd, 1941).

In the South, on the other hand, the land was in ruins. Small economic gains from before the war had vanished. Communities were destitute and unstable, and farmlands lay idle. Malaria was widespread. It would be another 20 years before a halting abatement of the disease in the South would be discernible (Faust, 1945).

Hungry People and Well-Fed Mosquitoes

Across the fertile bottomlands of the East Coast of the southern Atlantic, the Gulf Coast and the Mississippi delta region — all places that had been cleared before the war — lay uncultivated and undrained. More mosquitoes were breeding close to human habitation and more people were too undernourished and weak to resist infection.

Southern plantations were in disarray, and food was in short supply. Before the war most southerners — black and white, poor and wealthy — ate well. There had always been plenty of wild game for the table, including rabbits, raccoons, birds and deer. But after the war, any game that was left in the countryside was safe. The victorious troops from the North had taken away all the guns.

Many of the rural people throughout the South abandoned the farms and moved to coastal cities where new acute disease problems emerged.

Boyhood Memories

One of the nation's leading pioneering malariologists learned as a boy the direct relationship between malaria and rural deprivation in the post Civil War South.

Henry Rose Carter wrote later about life on the family plantation at the end of the war. In land, his father was rich. The plantation covered about 1,600 acres. But acreage cleared and drained before the war lay overgrown, and ditches were filled up. Living conditions were hard, as Carter remembered.

"There was a great increase of malaria after the Civil War in my section of Virginia — just above the Tidewater. This country had never been free from malaria; but on our plantation, at least, it had not been of sanitary importance for a number of years.[1] After the war several of the family had it — I and two little sisters — and it was fairly general, though not severe, all over our neighborhood.

...Take your choice as to the weight of the different factors (that favored survival of the disease). We thought — and I still think — that the abandonment of the land, and especially of the bottomland, leading to poor drainage, was the most important...

From the time Sheridan went through, in April 1865, we had no meat of any kind — save a few birds and two rabbits that we boys killed with stones — until November 18, when we killed a wild hog, a descendant of tame ones, in a trap. We had a little flour, and our family lived practically on partially spoilt corn (that is, the 'nubbin pile' — all the rest had been taken), potatoes, and wild salad plants, especially watercress" (Barber, 1929).[2]

As clearing and planting resumed, malaria gradually disappeared, retreating eastward toward the coast. Wheat was a profitable cash crop in Carter's area, but not for long. Soon new farms in Minnesota and the Dakotas in the country's Northwest began to dominate the nation's wheat market, leaving many southern farmers destitute again. Drainage was neglected, and malaria rose once more.

Patterns of Restoration

More setbacks lay ahead, as the region crept toward economic stability. A common pattern emerged. After land was cleared and re-occupied, small community projects were launched. Typically, a gristmill was created, or a stream was impounded for electric power generation, a municipal water works was built, and roads improved. But the improvements at first created new pools of water that attracted new mosquito populations. When folks from surrounding areas arrived to take advantage of the improvements, they brought new strains of malaria in their blood. Fresh epidemics of malaria followed.

Many of the new folks then moved away, and improvements that had attracted them were abandoned. But more outsiders kept coming in, and the expanding improvements gradually provided stable growth.

The pattern was repeated, a tidal fluctuation of economic recovery measured by recurring disease that was common in underdeveloped endemic regions all over the world. The ravished South was full of examples, large and small.

Immigration swelled in the lower Mississippi Valley, for instance, straining resources and spreading disease. Finally, in the 1890s, the Mississippi River Commission in New Orleans built a levee system to drain the rich alluvial plains, expanding economic opportunities. That, of course, attracted more outsiders.

First, a resurgence of malaria struck the newly developed region. Then the disease receded and the recovery took hold — until the next wave of immigration threatened the stability. And on and on.

Measuring Malaria

How bad was malaria, really? It had always been a difficult disease to quantify. The Army statistics were helpful. But the best indications of the scope and severity of the disease were believed to be the considerable observations of people in the stricken communities. They included the visiting doctors who were building a body of common wisdom and empirical observations that eventually led to successful control strategies (Faust, 1945).

One of the frequent visitors to remote malarious locations was Dr. Henry Rose Carter. The boy from the plantation just above the Tidewater in Virginia received a medical degree from the University of Maryland in 1879 and devoted his long career to understanding and controlling malaria and yellow fever.

Carter said that in endemic regions of the South, 90 percent of the population had malaria each year. He said that compared with other diseases, "malaria stands first on the list for the injury it does to the community" (Carter, 1919).

Carter said many authorities didn't appreciate how bad malaria was. The reason was that malaria was a disease of rural poor people. Health authorities were focusing more on urban health.

Another reason that many people were unaware of the problems of malaria was that stricken communities were so used to it. It was expected that young people would have chills and fever off and on in the early years of their lives, until they acquired some limited immunity. Those children, Carter said, were handicapped during the years of their growth and schooling (Ibid.). And, of course, a lot of children didn't live long enough to grow up. Their exposure to malaria left them particularly vulnerable to other diseases in their communities.

Investigating a mystery

Differences were widening between the two big reservoirs of malaria, the South and the Midwest, also known as the upper Mississippi River Basin. By the year 1875 the great migrations into the Midwest had ended, and the malaria prevalence there began a steep drop.

Some people referred to that reversal as a "mysterious" retreat. "Mysterious" because there was no single apparent reason for the disappearance, though there was no shortage of theories. The retreat came without any big public health campaigns to control it or any new medicines or treatments that people usually associated with victory over disease. The retreat came even before anyone knew that the mosquito was the vector.

A clear picture of the malaria retreat in the Midwest came many years later. In the 1940s, a historian published a comprehensive review of documents, letters, interviews, medical journals and personal correspondence about factors that might have accounted for the disappearance of the disease. Edwin Ackerknecht, an immigrant from the Netherlands, compiled lists of the reasons or clues offered by informed people. The tips led him to an assortment of theories and observations, which he cross-referenced and checked all across the Midwest.

Everywhere he looked, Ackerknecht's goal was focused. He wanted an answer to one burning question: what caused the abrupt reversal of malaria in the upper Mississippi River Basin, where the disease had been so pervasive for such a long time?

He reviewed his information, discarding factors that seemed to relate to conditions or events after the collapse of the disease had already begun. Some suggestions seemed to reflect a consequence of the drop in malaria instead of a cause. Some of the facts offered were so intertwined in the structure of the communities that it was hard to distinguish with precision what really had an effect on the dynamics of the health of the region.

Historian's List

At last Ackerknecht narrowed his list to five factors that combined to evict the disease, and he ranked them in importance:
The End of the Migration: No new strains were entering the area to stoke transmission of the disease. A report of the Malaria Commission of the League of Nations in 1927 had described that phenomenon. "Nothing is more favorable to high inci-

dence and severity of malaria than frequent movements of a population hither and thither in search of a bare living or of a place where the conditions of life are less hard, and very few things have a greater effect in reducing malaria than the stability of the population which comes when such a place is found" (Ackerknecht, 1945).

The Coming of the Railroad: The railroad replaced waterways as choice locations for settlement. First, the digging of the rail beds created pools and ditches where mosquitoes could breed. Localized increases of malaria followed, but those problems quickly disappeared. By the mid-1850s most people in the Midwest were settling by the new railroads instead of by the waterfront, thus reducing their proximity to breeding mosquitoes.

Drainage: Evaluating the effect of draining the countryside was a challenge to the historian. Natural drainage occurred everywhere that land was plowed and planted. Most of the big public drainage programs for agricultural development took place after malaria was already in retreat. But Ackerknecht's research convinced him that systematic drainage might have been particularly important in the disappearance of the disease in long-suffering Illinois. As it had already happened in Europe, drainage programs in places where the natural environment had been disrupted permitted farmers better profits from their land. Then came prosperity, which never did tolerate malaria.

Improved Housing: The conversion from log cabins to frame houses also helped suppress malaria. Several doctors in Ackerknecht's survey reported that log cabins were unhealthy, mainly because they gave mosquitoes easy entry. By 1860, half the rural population in the United States still lived in log cabins, especially common along the streams of Illinois. In many frontier towns, the doctor was the first one in the community to build himself a frame house. For the farmer, folks figured it took him four to seven years to earn enough from his new crops to convert from logs to frame *(Ibid.)*. And that frame house was usually quite a distance from the riverbanks. The historian concluded that screening actually wasn't an important contributor to the solution of the mystery. He said people in the Midwest didn't get screens for doors and windows until later.

Livestock: That factor was fascinating. The introduction of livestock was particularly important in evicting malaria from Wisconsin, Iowa and Minnesota. As farmers in Europe had noticed earlier, some mosquitoes that had a choice would rather take their blood meals from farm animals than from people. Farmers who lived in frame houses and kept livestock in barns close to the house got some relief from malaria. Presumably those mosquitoes had easier access to the livestock. Rural people eventually had enough resources to build barns, often with haylofts, which created a convenient retreat for mosquitoes.

One curious, well-traveled doctor said, "I have often seen thousands of *A. Quadrimaculatus* (a common species of *Anopheles* mosquito) in stables of that type situated in the prairie rice country of Arkansas" (Barber, 1929). It was observed that the dark corners of the barn were popular resting-places for exhausted mosquitoes. They needed a safe hiding place, according to one theory, almost as much as they needed warm blood to feed on. Mosquitoes were practically immobilized and vulnerable after they sucked up two and one-half times their body weight in blood. Several consultants to Ackerknecht thought this cattle-barrier was the only "naturalist" method of malaria control that showed enough promise to be promoted on a wide scale (Ackerknecht, 1945).

The dairy industry shifted from New England to the Midwest in the 1850s. That was fortunate for Wisconsin, whose previously prosperous wheat production was plagued by rust. In the last days of the Civil War, cheese was bringing a high price, so Wisconsin farmers switched to dairy production. Then the state became malaria-free. Some mosquitoes reportedly liked American horses, too. The famous Pennsylvania doctor Benjamin Rush wrote in 1797, "In Philadelphia, fevers are less known in the neighborhood of livery stables than in any other part of the city" *(Ibid.).*

More Issues

Two additional factors were mentioned frequently by Ackerknecht's informants. They were climate and quinine. Malaria might not have retreated so quickly if the region had been warmer. "Temperature is a very important element in the continuance of the process," said the historian. The parasite needed several months of warm weather to beat the tremendous mathematical odds against ongoing transmission.

A large group of infected people residing near an immense number of mosquitoes was required to keep the disease vital. In places where the warm season was short, the odds were even more stacked against the disease. Thus, malaria in the North required larger groups of infected people to keep the mosquito-parasite-humankind cycle intact.[3]

On the quinine issue, the historian concluded that the medicine had only an indirect effect on the disease. He drew on the better understanding of quinine in later years. Quinine did not cure malaria. It merely relieved those debilitating symptoms, at least temporarily. Even after the symptoms disappeared, the infected person still had malaria parasites in his or her blood. A mosquito could still remove those disease organisms along with its blood meal. Then, the mosquito could inject the disease into somebody else when it was ready to eat again.

In fact, doctors came to realize that quinine deprived the sick person of any immunity he or she may have received from the infection. The victim would be like a nonimmune the next time the disease struck. Re-infection was common.

In a way, that's just what happened to the farmers of the Midwest. Quinine could make them feel good enough a great deal of the time to tend to their crops. Then when the cold months came, the farmer could build up his strength again for the next season of malaria. But the disease kept spreading until mosquitoes lost their breeding places close to where folks lived.

Ackerknecht did believe quinine was helpful, but indirectly. Without periodic relief from their agony, farmers might not have been able to carry on. But carry on they did. They were people with a good record for endurance. They had endured hardships of poor regions of Europe, congested city life in the East, and the dangerous, arduous trip West. After they found free empty land to till, many could survive with the expectation that a better life lay ahead.

Perhaps one more factor could be put on Ackerknecht's list. That was the tenacity of the frontier people.

Yellow Fever Gets the Headlines

While malaria was quickly disappearing in the Midwest without the help of targeted control programs, malaria in the South maintained its virulence and its low profile. But the disease soon would attract the attention of some influential people with a commitment to help. Malaria came in the back door at a turning point in American history.

The pivotal period in the South was at the turn of the 20th century. The issues were yellow fever, widescale unemployment and migration, a thirst for economic recovery, an expansion in international trade in fruit and sugar cane, a threat of revolution in Cuba, an activist U.S. press and, at last, discoveries of the mosquito's role as a disease vector.

Yellow fever, like malaria, was carried by its own specific family of mosquitoes that entered the U.S. as stowaways. Many used to regard yellow fever as the urban version of malaria, the disease of rural poor. But they were two distinct diseases, and understanding the differences as well as the similarities would illuminate some of the problems people encountered in trying to control each of them.

The diseases were far more different than similar. Like malaria, yellow fever made people acutely sick with fever and pain. Yellow fever also caused internal hemorrhage, vomiting of thick black blood, jaundice that turned the skin yellow and convulsions leading to coma and death. Yellow fever caused more alarm, but malaria took more lives (Warner, 1989).

Yellow fever struck port cities and only infrequently, in violent, unpredictable epidemics. Several years might pass before the next eruption. On the other hand, most of the malaria in the U.S. was endemic. It settled down in an underdeveloped community and stayed a long time. Malaria inflicted its worst damage on children under five. Yellow fever mostly chose active adults and men more than women. Young children and old people may have been endowed with some inherent immunity to the disease.

The malaria parasite was a member of one of the oldest groups of animal organisms, the protozoa. It was so biologically integrated with the immune system of its human host that neither medicines nor vaccines seemed to control or prevent it, at least not by the end of the 20th century. People could get malaria over and over. Yellow fever was a virus and comparatively easy to control with a vaccine. A person who survived yellow fever was immune for life. Both diseases cost their communities dearly.

Yellow fever precipitated widespread panic. Big port cities receiving shipments of food products from tropical places were struck by the disease at least once. New Orleans, the old city on the Mississippi River delta on the Gulf of Mexico, was the most vulnerable by far. The city had more people than it could accommodate. From 1840 to 1855, half a million immigrants landed from Ireland and Germany to live in New Orleans. Then, at the end of the Civil War, the city continued to swell with the arrival of freed slaves from all over the South. New Orleans, known for its promise as a shipping hub for trade with Latin America, was the only city in the South that was thriving. Trade with Latin America was one of the most vital new industries in the country. U.S. investments in Cuba were estimated at $50,000,000. The annual U.S. trade with Cuba was estimated at $100,000,000.

In spite of its prosperity, New Orleans also was becoming notorious for its health hazards. The city had virtually no safe water, or plumbing, or sufficient shelter, or jobs. Health providers, civic leaders, church figures, business people and the vociferous daily press all lobbied government officials for sanitation reform and public health facilities. By the time it became clear that yellow fever was being brought to New Orleans in fruit boats from Cuba and other places, the passionate constituency for public health reform turned up the volume.

In Washington, D.C., some high-level people, including President William McKinley's personal physician Maj. Gen. Leonard Wood called for an invasion of Cuba. It was the only way to keep the U.S. safe from yellow fever, they argued. McKinley resisted the pressure, at least for a while.

The worst epidemic in New Orleans came in 1878, not without warning. U.S. shipping interests were advised that Cuba was suffering from an epidemic of a particularly deadly strain of yellow fever, and a cargo ship from that island was heading for New Orleans.

Quarantine facilities were alerted to tighten their scrutiny of debarking passengers and crew, but authorities then were not aware that mosquitoes carried the disease or that infected and contagious people would appear normal while the disease was incubating. Soon after passengers and crew debarked and the ship was unloaded, New Orleans was attacked by yellow fever. The disease exceeded its usual boundaries, pushing out of the congested, unsanitary, waterfront quarters and into residential neighborhoods of the well-to-do.

Panicked people were fleeing. The business community feared for the future of the city. Health professionals and volunteers were mobilized. The Public Health Service organized emergency shelters and treatment centers. Sick people were isolated. An estimated 6,000 people died, a figure that represented an estimated 20 to 70 percent of people with full-blown disease.

Then, just as it had happened with previous epidemics of yellow fever, the disease subsided. With good nursing care, most of the infected people would have a full recovery and then lifetime immunity (Ellis, 1992).

Meanwhile, business people, the press and politicians persisted in their demands for U.S. action against Cuba to force a public health cleanup.[4]

Spanish-American War

While New Orleans was recovering from its most devastating epidemic of yellow fever, an internal political crisis in Cuba gained momentum. By 1895, an insurgency of native Cubans had reached the intensity of a civil war for independence from Spain. It was the second installment of a two-part rebellion against Spain, whose overseas empire had brought it so much wealth and glory.

Rebels attacked government buildings as well as farms and businesses owned by the well-to-do Spanish rulers or by other members of the wealthy elite. The Spanish forces filled the jails with insurgents and confined others in large open-air "reconstruction" areas, reportedly with virtually no food, shelter, sanitation, or medical attention. Thousands of the detained people reportedly died of exposure, hunger and disease (Harrison, 1978; Britannica, 1965; Thomas, 1998).

Public opinion in the U.S. sympathized with the insurgents, as victims of abusive and autocratic European rulers. It was a familiar chord. The press was indignant, especially the easily excited Pulitzer newspaper *The New York World* and the important Hearst paper *The New York Journal*. Reports of the suffering of the captive activists were front-page fare, with large black headlines and graphic cartoon illustrations. The Commander of the Spanish forces, Gen. Valeriano Weyler y Nicolau, was nicknamed "the Butcher." That kind of journalism won the papers the sobriquet, the "yellow press." As attacks accelerated between the insurgents and Spanish defense forces, McKinley reportedly was close to dropping his reluctance to intervene. Dramatic events followed in rapid sequence.

In December 1897, new riots erupted in Havana, and the U.S. battleship Maine was dispatched to Havana harbor to stand by to protect U.S. property and evacuate U.S. citizens, if necessary. On February 15, 1898, the Maine sank in an explosion, killing 260 personnel. Based on the common assumption that the explosion was a deliberate act of aggression, the U.S. lobbying for war intensified. Theodore Roosevelt, assistant secretary of the Navy, said McKinley "has no more backbone than a chocolate éclair" (Thomas, 1998). The slogan "Remember the Maine — the hell with Spain" survived historically until the 1970s when the real story of the sinking of the Maine was brought to light. The explosion had been an accident.[5]

On March 17, McKinley gave up his reluctance to invade and sent an ultimatum to Madrid. It asked Spain to abandon its reconstruction program, declare an armistice and enter peace negotiations with the insurgents. The answer was ambiguous, and insurgents intensified their attacks. Then Madrid took the lead, declaring war on the U.S., and the U.S. Congress responded with its own declaration of war dated April 21.

The first engagement of the Spanish-American War was not in Cuba, but at Manila Bay in Spain's sprawling colony in the Pacific, the Philippine Islands. A squadron of the U.S. Asiatic naval force arrived from Hong Kong. Before dawn on May 1, and under Commodore George Dewey, the U.S. ships destroyed the enemy ships anchored in the harbor.

Dewey detailed a small unit of troops to occupy the city. A

larger U.S. force of 11,000 arrived in the Philippines by the end of July, and on August 13 they took over Manila. The hostilities were practically bloodless.[6]

The victory in Cuba was almost as easy for the U.S., basically another naval victory. A Spanish fleet of four armored cruisers and three destroyers arrived off Santiago on the southern shores of Cuba to protect the island. American naval forces blockaded the entrance and followed the Spanish ships up the coast. On land near Santiago, a U.S. force including a volunteer unit called the Rough Riders engaged defending forces in two battles, at El Caney and then at San Juan Hill (Britannica, 1965).

Resistance was minimal. The defenders were defeated, but reports said the local malaria was an awesome menace. Perhaps the most lasting historic image of the engagement was the victory photograph: U.S. troops posed on the top of San Juan Hill. The U.S. flag waved overhead, and in the foreground was Theodore Roosevelt, commander of the unit of volunteers.

He had several reasons to be proud. As assistant secretary of the Navy, Roosevelt was credited with the achievement of keeping all U.S. ships well-equipped, trained and ready for action in the right place at the right time.

The coup de grace of the war was a naval engagement in which the U.S. sank all the Spanish ships off Cuba, except for the ones left burning or in sinking condition.

An armistice was signed on August 12, less than four months from the original declaration of war. Negotiations for the final settlement came December 10.

Historians said McKinley had expected to acquire only Manila in the Pacific, as well as Cuba. But advisers convinced him that the new naval victories had proven the U.S. deserved and needed the whole package, the entire archipelago of the Philippines with an estimated 7,000 islands inhabited by seven million people. The U.S. victors got that and more. The settlement included the islands of Guam and Puerto Rico. In total, a huge bounty for a little war.

A Pivotal Discovery

On the other side of the world, in colonial India, a British Army medical officer, Ronald Ross, was making history alone in his lab. He discovered in September 1897 that mosquitoes carry malaria, and that led to the discovery three years later that a different genus of mosquitoes also carries yellow fever. He obviously understood the vast significance of his discovery when he wrote a poem that night:

> "This day relenting God,
> Hath placed within my hand
> A wondrous thing; and God
> Be praised. At his command
> Seeking his secret deeds
> With tears and toiling breath
> I find thy cunning seeds.
> O million murdering death."

Now the world was capable of rationally controlling its most deadly disease. Malaria was preventable.

Cuba and Panama

The United States was a world power with territorial interests on two oceans. Within days after Roosevelt stood with the flag on San Juan Hill, McKinley gave the job as governor of Cuba to his personal physician General Wood, and gave the job as director of yellow fever eradication to another U.S. Army physician, Major George Gorgas. Gorgas, a southerner, had volunteered for the job because he once had yellow fever, leaving him immune for life.

His associates in Cuba included Major Walter Reed, who had just proven yellow fever was carried by mosquitoes,[7] Dr. Henry Rose Carter, whose childhood and career were dominated by the challenges of mosquito-borne diseases, other prominent

74

scientists, sanitation engineers and military figures. They all could assume, rightfully, that the U.S. government would spend whatever the job required.

First, Gorgas divided Havana into zones. Every zone was inspected regularly. Every property owner was held responsible for eliminating mosquito breeding on his or her own property. Every resident had to empty all water containers on his property, and use screens, oils, or larvicides where needed. The fine for people who didn't comply was $10.00.

The *Aedes aegypti* mosquitoes that transmitted yellow fever thrived in cities, where compliance with control regulations was easy. Gorgas seemed to work the hardest. Often he was seen late in the afternoon walking alone, conducting his own personal inspection (Harrison, 1978). It wasn't hard to spot the places where *Aedes* bred. They weren't shy, not like the *Anopheles*. They could even breed in an abandoned vase in the bedroom.

Gorgas had money left over from his budget to press on into the outskirts of the territory where the anophelines that carried malaria bred in their own favorite settings, in quiet water sheltered by dense vegetation. Malaria was widespread and not so easy to deal with. That was mainly the job of J. A. LePrince, who became well known for his work later in Panama and the U.S. South. Both diseases were presumed evicted from Cuba by 1902.

Logical Next Step

After the U.S. proclaimed victory over oppression and disease in Cuba, appeals for further international expansion were hard to resist. The new president made it easier. He was Theodore Roosevelt, who was vice president when President McKinley was killed by an assassin's bullet on September 6, 1901.

Roosevelt was an expansionist, fully supporting the idea that the country's new Pacific possessions needed to be protected, and international business interests needed help competing with European traders who had a head start doing business with Asia.

Even religious missions were pressing for chances to expand into Asia. The next step seemed logical — dig a canal to link the two big oceans.

France had tried in 1879 to dig a canal through the Isthmus of Panama. That team gave up after 10 years. Actually, they were defeated, defeated by disease. Malaria and yellow fever were indeed horrible. The death rate among canal workers in that failed mission was 63.1 per 1000 (Harrison, 1978, p. 163).

As the U.S. excavation and construction crews began their work, Gorgas set out with his own team to accompany Army engineers and lead the battle against yellow fever. He expected, and rightly so, that he could count on at least some of the team from the Cuba project to join him and count on all the money and support he needed from the U.S. government. He could count on all the new information from entomologists who kept revealing new minute details about the behavior of the two villain vectors: *Anopheles,* which transported malaria in the rural areas, and *Aedes,* which transported yellow fever in the two terminal cities, Balboa and Colon.

But Gorgas did not count on how difficult it would be to control malaria. The entire campaign against both diseases took 10 years, 1904–14. The more accommodating yellow fever was virtually eradicated by 1906, when only one case was reported. LePrince was in charge of controlling the recalcitrant malaria.

The new canal was designed to follow the 47-mile path of the old railroad. The work force of 80,000 engineers and laborers dragged heavy excavation equipment as they lurched through the tropical jungle, digging, draining swamps, clearing thick vegetation and leaving countless ponds and depressions where mosquitoes could breed. The workers lived in 30 villages and camps along the way, mostly close to the water's edge. Many of them slept in tents or temporary barracks. Some of the crew had immunity to malaria and some did not.

In the beginning, the incidence of malaria was more than 800 per 1000 workers. The crews and supervisors experimented along the way, creating their own protection. They developed ditching strategies, made mosquito nets and created larvicides. One of the new larvicides, Paris Green, was an arsenic compound subsequently used for many years with success all over the world. By 1916, malaria incidence was down to 15 per 1000.

The malaria protection for the Panama Canal cost $3 million, or $3.50 per person protected in the 100-square-mile control project (*Ibid.* p. 167). It made malaria protection appear beyond the reach of most state or county budgets in the U.S. But visiting specialists from Europe were impressed by what they saw and based projects in their own countries or colonies on the Panama strategies. The two successful campaigns, Panama and Cuba, opened a prominent professional niche for many years to come for American and European malariologists and sanitation engineers.

---

[1] "Sanitary" was commonly used to describe conditions that influenced public health. "Sanitarian" referred to physicians or public health workers who specialized in establishing or maintaining conditions that protected a community's health. They became the front-line of defense against malaria.

[2] Carter's recollections were in a letter he wrote to M. A. Barber in 1925, the year of his death.

[3] See 'Slim odds for transmission' on p. 117 for a discussion of the variables that regulate malaria transmission.

[4] England was ahead of the U.S. in modernizing city services to protect citizens from disease. Epidemics of infectious diseases were common in London and other principal cities during the Industrial Revolution, which attracted large-scale influx of poor people from rural areas. Following the cholera epidemic of 1849, London created a comprehensive public health act. It was a model for large cities everywhere (Learmonth, 1988).

5 U.S. Admiral Hyman Rickover, Commander of the U.S. nuclear submarine fleet, conducted a long enquiry of the incident. His conclusion, "How the Battleship Maine was Destroyed," was published by the Naval History Division, Department of the Navy, 1976. The explosion that destroyed the ship was set off by heat from an accidental fire in a coalbunker adjacent to the reserve magazine (Thomas, 1998).

6 The U.S. occupation of the Philippines yielded lessons about malaria control. The Army, long aware of the health hazards in swampy areas, erected most of its barracks in the hills near open running water. But that part of Asia was populated by an aggressive mosquito vector that favored a highland habitat and sunny streams. Malaria was common. The *Anopheles* species breeding in dark lowland marshes near the waterfront were harmless. Troops billeted there stayed well (Herms, 1940).

7 Several sources gave credit for the discovery to Carlos Finlay of Havana. He had released his findings in 1881. Reed, a bacteriologist, was head of the U.S. Army Yellow Fever Commission. He verified Finlay's conclusions in 1900 with experiments using human volunteers, some of whom sacrificed their lives (Britannica, 1965).

Chapter 4

Golden Age of Malariology

IN SPITE OF ALL the new lessons about mosquito vectors and control techniques, a range of specific malaria trouble spots persisted. In the U.S. Northeast, small, localized epidemics were squelched, thanks to the new knowledge about the transmission process. Two urban campaigns were notable.

In 1901, alarming reports of a malaria epidemic reached the health office of the Port of New York. The site was an area of Staten Island under development and heavily populated by vector mosquitoes. The successful control campaign was remembered as the first big city antimalaria project making use of the new knowledge of the mosquito's role in delivering and perpetuating the disease.

The project was led by Alvah H. Doty, health officer of the Port of New York. In his initial investigation, Doty visited one section of a community where mosquitoes were particularly dense. One-fifth of the inhabitants were infected with the disease. In one house alone, he found 22 mosquitoes, about half of which were anopheline. A sick person was lying in a corner in the grips of an acute attack of malaria.

Health officers located swamps along the coast where the mosquitoes bred, and the land was reclaimed. Crews dug almost 1,000 miles of drainage canals at a cost of $50,000, and by 1909 malaria was virtually gone. Only five cases were reported, not enough to permit ongoing transmission in that setting (Matheson, 1941; Russell, 1943, p 620; Harrison, 1978, p 168).

In retrospect, some specialists criticized Doty's strategy. Critics pointed out that trying to exterminate all mosquitoes in a malarious region was a waste of resources. The job would have been a lot easier and cheaper if it primarily focused on the elimination of contact points between specific communities of mosquito vectors and very sick malaria victims. The Staten Island strategy seemed extravagant to some specialists who believed they were making progress on creating cost-effective control solutions (Boyd, 1941).

The response a few years later to a malaria epidemic in Ithaca, N.Y., was an example of a more sharply focused strategy. The specialists identified the victims, found the specific breeding areas of the vectors, and tried to eliminate them. The disease in Ithaca still took a long time to control.

The Ithaca outbreak was in 1904. (Coincidentally, it came just a year after the town was hit by a typhoid epidemic.) Nearly 2,000 malaria cases were reported in the population of 13,000. All the city's doctors were required to report every week on the details of each case, including the results of blood examinations and the locations where each victim lived or was bitten.

An inspector and two assistants located specific mosquito breeding places among the cattail marshes on three sides of the city. Townspeople were taught how malaria was contracted and how to avoid infection. People also were instructed to isolate patients so mosquitoes could not bite the human carriers and thus spread the infection to others.

Meanwhile, city workers treated the marshes for six years with kerosene oil every week or 10 days, preventing the establishment of new mosquito nurseries close to where people lived. In one year, the number of infected people was cut in half, down to 1,000. By 1908 there were none (Matheson, 1941).

In California, several creative programs were initiated to solve particular mosquito problems in the Pacific Coast salt marshes. The first of those programs was in Burlingame, California, in 1905. Then in 1910, the first mosquito abatement program for controlling malaria in an endemic area in the U.S. was conducted in Penryn, California. In 1912 the first malaria-mosquito abatement program at an irrigation district in the U.S. was installed at Los Molinos, California (Herms, 1940).

Unlike in the South, thriving communities in the North and in California obviously had money and other resources for thorough, aggressive public health programs.

Problems Linger in South

In the South, malaria was still much worse than in the North. But new attention from outside sources was coalescing and creating an effective constituency for disease control. Money and help were on the way.

Malariologists home from Panama and Cuba had new lessons to share from their hands-on experiences. And they had an ever-growing bank of new knowledge from entomologists about the mosquito's role in transmission. They had new support from public officials who had watched with horror the mayhem caused by yellow fever, and support also from the country's business community and its philanthropy.

Forging Links

Back home from his work in Panama, Henry Rose Carter linked with the newly invigorated Public Health Service, and with state and local health providers to design cost-effective, community-based malaria protection. Carter always seemed to have an eye on costs. He estimated that more than $100 million already had been spent on improvements critical in early stages of economic development. Those included shoreline reclamation, dams, stream diversion, power stations and road construction. Invariably the improvements were invitations for mosquitoes. Carter figured another $100 million or more would be needed in the future.

Starting in 1913, Carter directed a Public Health Service series of malaria control demonstrations in Mississippi, North Carolina and Virginia. Teams analyzed specific trouble spots, trying to create low-cost solutions that could be installed and maintained by local authorities under the guidance and minimal support from state and county public health staff. Project managers were shown ways to anticipate future malaria problems before construction began (Carter, 1919).

Rockefeller Joins the Initiative

During the same period but under different names, the Rockefeller Foundation was creating malaria education and prevention projects in endemic areas. The Foundation had long been sensitive to the relationship between chronic disease and tangible profits at factories in the South. Workers there were not nearly so productive as workers in the North.

The Foundation sent teams to the South to study the problem.[1] They concluded that the low productivity was due to widespread, debilitating hookworm. The Rockefeller experts controlled that disease and production improved. Later the Foundation took on yellow fever, finally creating a successful vaccine against that disease. Then the Foundation directed its attention to the problems of malaria.

The Rockefeller Foundation joined the malaria control programs in the South in 1916, linking with the Department of

Health in Mississippi and the Public Health Service in Arkansas. The project was extensive, including the creation of large hydroelectric installations, extensive drainage projects and rice culture programs.

Public health consultants helped construction engineers before their work started, identifying, for instance, places on the periphery of a future dam where a spillover was a possibility. Overflows around impoundments frequently created isolated spills where mosquitoes bred. Often a construction team worked with the health consultants in planning ways to treat the bottoms of impoundments or ditches to inhibit growth of vegetation that would be particularly attractive to *Anopheles* mosquitoes.

The health teams also helped certain factory managers figure out why so many of their workers were getting malaria. One grateful mill owner wrote to Carter about the miller's experience. He said, "The money spent in your campaign against malaria here gave the quickest and most enormous returns I have ever known from any investment." The cost for improvements for malaria control was 80 cents per worker for the first year and 27 cents for the second year. The result was a rise in mill efficiency from 50 percent to normal.

Public health teams also consulted state and county authorities in creating requirements for malaria protection in building plans. Sometimes details of an approved plan were ignored, and the new facility did in fact attract anophelines that spread malaria. The project then might be cited for responsibility of any new outbreak of disease. That had happened in litigation in 1913 against developers of the Hales Bar impoundance project on the Tennessee River.

Lessons for Everyone

Sometimes the visiting health workers and engineers themselves learned important lessons from the project managers, often with far-reaching implications. Carter wrote about a new impoundment to generate power for a cotton mill at Baleswetts Falls in a malarious region of North Carolina. The power plant was shut down every Saturday at noon until Monday morning. The 42 hours of downtime allowed the water to rise 24 inches or so. After the weekend, when demand for power resumed, the water level fell fast. The same thing happened to a lesser degree every evening when there was less demand for power, thus less demand for water. The following morning the level rose slightly.

Malaria at that particular location was no problem. The reason was simple. The minor turbulence on the surface of the pond disturbed the mosquito larvae floating and feeding on the surface. The larvae required about 10 days of still water to complete their feeding and maturation. The new observations at the small installation were decisive later in designing large-scale projects elsewhere in the U.S. and worldwide.

Meanwhile, local citizenry were learning basic lessons about how to distinguish potential malaria vectors from all the other mosquito colonies in their region. Malaria was carried only by certain species of the *Anopheles* genus, and that genus had at least two characteristics that anyone could see. When an anopheline came to rest on the arm of the selected victim, it tilted its body head down at about a 45-degree angle. Other mosquitoes stayed poised parallel to the surface. There were other differences. When the anopheline larvae lay resting and feeding on surface minutiae in sheltered still water, they floated just under the surface and parallel to it. Other mosquitoes attached themselves to the surface of the water by a breathing device on their anterior. They fed head down on various substances floating on the water (Herms, 1940).

Poor regions in the South already beginning to experience some prosperity and some relief from malaria got a new boost from the U.S. government. The Army began construction of 43 barracks and other projects in 15 states in the South. The Public Health Service developed malaria control projects at each place, providing more awareness about disease prevention and providing more jobs and buying power for local people. Southerners no longer had to migrate north to get a good job.

Public Health Strategies

In World War I (1914–1918), much of Europe was devastated, and the toll of emotionally and physically wounded was incalculable. But when soldiers infected with malaria started returning home, a new trend became apparent in the United States. It was less likely that the malaria they brought with them from the battle zones would be transmitted to other people in their home communities. Less likely, that is, than after previous wars (Carter, 1919).[2]

After World War I, national and international interest in malaria was heightened. Several American malaria specialists took part in recovery programs in Europe sponsored by the Rockefeller Foundation and the League of Nations Malaria Commission.

Within the United States the disease continued as a public health problem in the South, but transmission decreased. People began to notice that well-defined zones of endemic malaria from the past were beginning to shrink, even in the presence of continued heavy populations of mosquitoes. Even in some locations where mosquitoes seemed to be more abundant than before, malaria was down.

Health authorities who regularly visited endemic areas were noticing that the infectious locations were becoming smaller around the edges. Malaria was shrinking like a melting snowball.

New micromanaged control strategies were installed, similar to the strategies used many years later in San Diego County to locate and eliminate communities of mosquitoes that were spreading malaria among migrant workers. Public health specialists were focusing on the periphery of malarious zones, linking sick individuals with mosquito communities that might be transmitting the disease. Then public health workers could eliminate the contact points where the vectors and the victims might be meeting. That disintegration of the transmission zone often left a remaining core of transmission that was incapable of sustaining itself, no matter how many mosquitoes were left in the neighborhood.

As it shrank beyond the historic cores of endemicity, malaria started a slow and bumpy retreat. Looking back, malaria specialists realized the disease had been well on its way to defeat even before the Public Health Service expanded its malaria programs. A natural momentum had begun, similar to the momentum that began in 1875 in the Midwest and quickly defeated malaria there.

New Regulations for Protection

More new development projects throughout the South incorporated malaria control regulations and guidelines, but sometimes the guidelines were ignored, with terrible consequences.

An epidemic broke out among residents close to the new Gantt Reservoir in Alabama, which was impounded without prior clearing to thwart mosquito breeding. When work began in 1922, 16 cases of malaria were recorded in a population of about 250.

It was demonstrated that the assigned construction firm had ignored the guidelines, convincing The U.S. Public Health Service to take steps later to enforce compliance with terms. On the advice of the Health Service, the State of Alabama passed regulations in 1923 and readopted them in 1927 to require detailed preparations before creation of impoundments. Other states followed Alabama's lead and set up their own regulations and policies for malaria control.

The Perennial Problem of Statistics

It was believed that national or state reporting methods were not consistent or reliable (Faust, 1941; Mountin, 1944). More credence was given to specific observations by health professionals who frequently visited rural endemic areas. One well-traveled doctor reported a 52 percent drop in cases in Mississippi within 10 years (Bass, 1927).

A survey in 1923–25 of irrigated rice regions in Arkansas and Louisiana showed that mosquitoes were abundant, but malaria had subsided to levels where it was no longer a health problem. The growers were becoming prosperous and had screens on their doors and windows (Barber, 1929). In 1928, in the Elsberry, Missouri, region where malaria was once a serious health problem, the disease had become rare. The mosquitoes, including the kind that carried the disease, were abundant, but the people were prospering and could protect themselves (*Ibid.*).

Health Care Bargains

County and community organizations joined in control projects, often improvising with cheap local products. Some creative people concocted their own larvicides, using among other things waste tobacco stems, tea, chrysanthemum flowers and bark from a variety of trees (LePrince, 1932).

In Shelby County, Tennessee, county commissioners sponsored several malaria control projects in the post-World War I period. People lined bottoms of flat-grade ditches with light concrete bottoms. They distributed insect-feeding minnows to stock 2,300 ponds, lakes and other still bodies of water. A new community industry collected crank case oil, separated it and stored it. The resulting light oil reportedly was effective in killing mosquito larvae. Local people also collected scrap sheet metal and disposable crate wood to make inexpensive screening for windows and doors for tenant farms.

In the late 1920s in LeFlore County, Mississippi, residents created an inexpensive model of screens that became widely popular as the "Public Health Service Door" (Watson and Maher, 1932, p. 655).

County home and farm agents organized projects for the citizenry, including school children. Prizes were awarded at the Mid-South Fair in Memphis for the best health projects (LePrince, 1932). One man even created a device for electrocuting mosquitoes as they flew in the window.

New scattered reports of the retreat or recurrences of the disease were recorded in letters or journals. In the late 1920s, isolated new outbreaks were noticed, attributed usually to exceptional flooding in 1927, and to the subsequent decline of cotton production. On balance, recovery was easy to explain. But the economic crash that was to follow stunned the entire country and created conditions that led to new epidemics of malaria.

The Great Depression

The Great Depression starting in 1929 brought a sharp reversal to the descending path of the disease. Financial institutions crashed. Factories were idled, and homeless people had to camp in parks and vacant lots. By 1932, the U.S. manufacturing output had dropped 54 percent from the 1929 level. Unemployment had risen to 25 or 30 percent of the work force. Misery was everywhere, especially in the South, where the important cotton industry was practically at a standstill (Grolier Encyclopedia Online, 1993). While the economy crashed, malaria transmission soared. One calculation put the number of malaria cases in the U.S. in 1932 at 1,500,000 and then the number of cases in 1934 at 2,700,000 (Herms, 1940).

Malaria control became one of the planks of the New Deal, President Roosevelt's program to crank up the economy and improve social services and health for the unemployed poor.

He created the WPA (Work Projects Administration) and CCC (Civilian Conservation Corp), staffing them from the ranks of the unemployed poor. A principal goal was malaria control. Thousands unemployed men were assigned to drainage projects in 250 counties that were in most need of help. Crews dug 33,655 miles of ditches and removed 544,414 acres of *Anopheles* breeding surfaces in 16 states in the Southeast (Williams, 1941). Techniques used were similar to the old strategies honed by the early settlers in the U.S. South, and recovery was fast. A steep decline in the disease was noticed in 1934-35 (Mountin, 1944).

Public Power and Public Health

The premier program for malaria control was created in a poor, highly endemic region in the southern state of Tennessee. The Tennessee River Basin drained 41,000 square miles in seven states in the southern U.S.. The basin received more rainfall each year than any other region of its size in the country (Bishop, 1937). In the early 1930s about 2 million people lived there, mostly poor tenant farmers who grew corn and cotton but had not yet begun to recover from the depression. The economy of the region was still in shambles. Malaria was endemic.

That was where President Roosevelt in 1933 unveiled one of the boldest projects in his economic recovery strategy. The Tennessee Valley would become a parkland of new industries, hydroelectric power generators, farms, food processing plants, lakeside recreation facilities and more. The Tennessee Valley Authority (TVA) would also be the location of new nitrate production facilities to break the U.S. dependency on Germany and Chile for nitrates, a critical need for a world power that might be facing another big war.[3]

The Planning Stage

Protection from malaria at TVA was addressed even before the construction began. The man picked to be the health manager first took one year of special training in malaria. He also surveyed the TVA terrain and reviewed successful projects of the past, including the early work in the South, and pioneering projects in Cuba and Panama. Another phase of his preparation was studying the fast-growing bank of knowledge about the *Anopheles* mosquito (Derryberry, 1953).

Generation of hydroelectric power was the first concern at TVA. The new water control system provided for an integrated chain of man-made lakes with a shoreline of more than 10,000 miles. All the rain that fell over the basin would be put to work. The plan was designed to control floods for the entire river basin, develop navigation, produce and market electric power. It would link nine main streams with navigational locks, and 23 tributaries. In all, 32 major dams were built.

All the dams were managed as a single unit, allowing for a precisely synchronized schedule for raising and lowering all water levels to prevent mosquitoes from breeding. The planners also designated specific techniques for anticipating overflow problems at future impoundment sites. Marginal depressions left by the construction were sculpted and connected throughout the system to provide a nearly complete drainage of the vast river network. Meetings were held with wildlife conservationists and biologists to protect the natural setting, including migration routes of birds and local fish. In addition, large areas were set aside for recreation. Agriculture and timber were developed, as well as mineral resources, leaving the region beautiful, prosperous and healthy.

Over the years, TVA specialists tried several kinds of insecticides and larvicides for treating and reshaping the waters' edges, but the overriding strategy was to find naturalistic approaches to inhibit mosquito breeding without toxic materials. Planners judged that approach to be safer and cheaper for human habitation (Bishop, 1937).

Many clinics were established in the region, making it possible to confine people with late-stage malaria, and to provide more health education programs. In addition, landlords of the tenant farms were encouraged to provide screening for houses and other safeguards to protect people from mosquitoes. Links were established between the TVA facilities and other health providers in the region to allow an integrated public health policy (Watson and Maher, 1939).

In 1934, in an area in northern Alabama where a TVA reservoir was under development, a house-to-house survey for malaria was conducted with blood slides of local people. Twenty to 60 percent of the residents tested positive for malaria for an overall average of 30 percent. By 1948, no indigenous malaria was reported.

Experienced health workers in the region were surveyed for opinions about the various factors responsible for the successful malaria control, and the answers were predictable: improved standard of living, education and elimination of sheltered, shallow water. Soon it was obvious: in the South, as elsewhere, prosperity and health were clearly linked.

More War Preparations

By the mid-1930s, government planners realized a new world war was coming. And the new war, it was believed, would be much more damaging to the U.S. than was World War I. Several depressed sites in the South were selected for military development. Vast areas formerly distinguished by unhealthy, untilled land and widescale unemployment were targeted for shipyards, airforce bases, factories, barracks and modern commercial enterprises. Builders, contractors and malariologists had all the government money they needed. The renovation of the South was part of the military defense strategy and budget.

Soon most of the idle land was cleared, and chronic unemployment was gone.

The Vanishing of Malaria

Doctors and community health workers were the first to notice the steep and steady drop in malaria transmission. It began in the U.S. South and picked up momentum in 1934 and 1935 (Mountin, 1944).

By about 1939 malariologists were noticing that in areas where the disease was active, it was shrinking to the point where it lost its vigor to sustain ongoing transmission. The disease was no longer considered a public health threat.

Meanwhile, American malariologists had already been accepting assignments from the Rockefeller Foundation and other agencies to create malaria control programs in countries where the disease was still a threat. The strategies and techniques were largely based on early, successful projects at TVA, the Panama Canal, and places in California and the South.

Back home in the U.S. South, new public money for malaria control was available from various government allocations for depression relief and for modernization of vast areas picked for new defense facilities (Duffy, 1992, pp. 168-9). The Public Health Service was granted $2,142,860 for malaria control.

Malariologists thought it ironic that the new money was granted for mosquito control and new chemical weapons while malaria was already being controlled (Hackett, 1941). The conventional wisdom of those pioneer malariologists favored the use of successful drainage techniques and preferred concentrating on specific locations where malaria could be prevented. The strategy was to interrupt contact between human habitats and mosquito breeding areas, mostly by diverting standing water through ditching, draining and weeding. Experience showed that malaria was easier to control with a shovel than with a spray gun, and a lot cheaper.

To create a durable record of successful programs of the past, several of the senior scientists in the country wanted to produce a comprehensive public presentation of the findings of the pioneer malariologists. The American Association for the Advancement of Science (AAAS) provided the forum, a Symposium on Human Malaria in Philadelphia, Pa., from December 30, 1940, to January 1, 1941.

Forty-five scientists contributed articles for publication in the proceedings. Topics covered a wide scope: the history of malaria functioning and life style of *P. vivax* and *P. falciparum*, behavior and needs of the mosquito vectors, with details about vectors active in the U.S., malaria and the community, quinine and other antimalarial medicine, immunity, control programs, water management and studies of the disease in Panama and the Caribbean. In addition to the AAAS book, many other publications were issued describing in detail the creation of successful, low-cost control programs in a variety of settings.

One of the most influential malaria experts at the forum, Mark F. Boyd, said the modern methods wasted money and "undoubtedly retarded the control of malaria" (Boyd, 1941).

Boyd was outspoken about several issues of his time saying, "students of modern medicine were but slightly if at all familiar with the older writers." He said modern students "thus fail to appreciate the substantial character of the contributions which have come down to us from the past." He also pointed out, "It is often difficult for the physician with modern training to grasp fully the significance of the older writers" *(Ibid.)*.

The year 1941 would have been a logical place to end a history of malaria in the United States. By then, the disease was no longer significant. Two events, however, disrupted the course of logic and overshadowed the significance of the accomplishments of the old-fashioned but successful southern doctors.

First, the United States was suddenly flung into World War II, preoccupying sensibilities everywhere for years.

The other overshadowing event was the discovery of the killing power of a new insecticide called DDT. The two events were related only by coincidence and by the fact that both complicated an orderly summation of the disappearance of malaria. Repercussions would challenge objective assessments.

A Shipment From Switzerland

In 1942, the Geigy Company exported 200 pounds of DDT insecticide spray from Switzerland to the Bureau of Entomology and Plant Quarantine in Orlando, Florida. The remarkable product was used first to control moths in woolen products in Europe, and later as a weapon against human body lice that carried typhus.[4]

The new insecticide was soon in great demand. Japanese forces had restricted export of a critical component of Rotenone, a popular insecticide that had been available from Malaysia (formerly Malaya) and Singapore. Also, shipment of the once popular insecticide pyrethrum from Kenya was unreliable. A new product that could kill insects on contact was seen as an important breakthrough in science and an important addition to the military arsenal.

Several reasons were advanced for the use of DDT against malaria in the United States:

- As a residual spray, it could eradicate the disease while its presence was at a low ebb.
- It could protect civilians against transmission from infected service personnel returning home soon, or so the sponsors believed.
- It could protect the domestic population from a new widespread wave of the disease that might occur if the U.S. suffered a big depression after the war.
- Regular strategies used for malaria control were considered too expensive for wide use.

Each of those justifications advanced for using the product in the U.S. was compromised by one glaring fact. Malaria was no longer a public health threat in the U.S.. At least some of those suggested reasons, however, must have had a ring of credibility. The public did in fact accept DDT and allowed technicians to spray it on the inside walls of their houses. The product already had been used in crop spraying and experimental aerial spraying at TVA.

After a short testing period, a 36-square-mile area of cotton country near Helena in Arkansas was chosen in 1944 for the first large-scale indoor household spraying program. A public health service team, with the help of two high school boys, sprayed the interior walls of every house in the test area, skipping every 25th house to use for comparisons. Ninety-five percent of the homes were "of tenant or sharecropper type, shotgun construction, newspaper-lined, inhabited by Negroes making only a marginal living" (Science News Letter, 1944). At the end of the program, the team reported a 94 percent reduction of live mosquitoes resting on the walls.

The project was expanded the following year in the "Extended Program for Malaria Control." Indoor walls of 400,000 houses were sprayed at locations closer to areas of military significance, like barracks, airfields and wartime factories. There, the team leaders were satisfied that the DDT was keeping mosquitoes away. Another more complicated test was done. It was called a Precipitin test, which required examination of the insects' stomachs to see if they contained a recent blood meal. Most of the mosquitoes captured indoors did not contain blood. That was interpreted to indicate that, in houses sprayed with DDT, fewer people were bitten by mosquitoes. Or perhaps it indicated that fewer insects that entered people's houses came out with a blood meal in their stomachs. Tests did not indicate how much malaria was transmitted or avoided. In other words, the capacity of DDT to prevent malaria was not established.

Even then, in one of the first spraying assignments, the project operators reported that mosquitoes were developing resistance to the insecticide and that resistance was accelerating with repeated applications.

Sources reported that none of those projects was based on evaluation of actual transmission of malaria (Langmuir, 1963).

World War II

The U.S. entry into the new world war began suddenly one Sunday morning in 1941 with a Japanese attack on the U.S. naval base at Pearl Harbor in Hawaii. The weapons were new and the delivery systems were new, but it was the same old malaria. As one historian said, "The success of military campaigns since history has been recorded often hinged on the presence of this disease rather than on tactics or military strength" (Ognibene and Barrett, 1982).

In the allied campaign for Sicily, for instance, 21,482 U.S. troops were hospitalized with malaria. A total of 17,375 were hospitalized for wounds received in combat.

In the opening years of the Pacific campaigns, Japanese invaders took over cinchona plantations in Java, depriving the Allied Forces of quinine — an event that accelerated the search for alternatives to quinine. Casualties from malaria in Asia and the Pacific were terrible. The highest rates of the disease were believed to have been in the China-Burma-India theater. In the famous U.S. infantry unit in Burma (now Myanmar) called Merill's Marauders, nearly every soldier had malaria during the 4-month campaign. Ten percent of the 3,000 men had to be evacuated from behind enemy lines. The unit was heroically successful, but was so ravaged by disease that it had to be disbanded (Shanks, 1991).

In another military theater, malaria apparently was decisive in the defeat of American and Philippine forces by Japanese invaders on Bataan Peninsula in the Philippines. The *New York Times* headline said, "Troops on Bataan Routed by Malaria" (*N.Y. Times*, 18 April 1942, p. 5).

Malaria and malnutrition stalked the defeated troops on their long march to Japanese prison camps. Those two maladies combined to take a heavy toll in the camps (Gillespie, 1963). Later that year, General MacArthur rushed troops to defend Buna, Papua New Guinea, from Japanese invaders. The casualties from malaria were crippling, according to one historian. MacArthur said, "This will be a long war if for every division I have facing the enemy I must count on a second division in Hospital with malaria and a third division convalescing from this debilitating disease" (Condon-Rall, 1991).

Later in the war, U.S. forces began recapturing Pacific Islands that were writhing with malaria. New strains of the disease had been left there by Japanese invaders, and new breeding places for mosquitoes were created by deforestation, bomb craters, hastily built roads and even abandoned foxholes. Before the U.S. assault forces landed, the beachheads were sprayed from the air with DDT.

Hero Status for DDT

Two years after the antagonists signed the peace treaty ending World War II, DDT was hailed for its wartime accomplishments and for the claim that it eradicated malaria in the United States. One DDT supporter summed up the status, saying, "The failure of post-war malaria outbreaks to develop after its (DDT's) use during the extended malaria control program was generally conceded to be convincing evidence of its efficacy in preventing transmission" (Andrews, 1951). It was an example of that not uncommon skewed logic described as "post hoc, ergo hoc," or "after that, because of that."

An Unusual Meeting

A new commitment to eradicate malaria worldwide with residual spraying of DDT was announced at the 4th Congress of Tropical Medicine and Malaria in Washington, D.C., in 1948. E. J. Pampana, who had been selected to head the malaria program of the soon-to-be installed World Health Organization, unveiled details of the novel new program assigning exclusive reliance on DDT for malaria control. He said the public would welcome the campaign. "There probably never was another public health measure," he said, "that could sell so well as residual spraying."

Pampana forecast the end of conventional control programs. "We do hope malaria will one day be eradicated from the world, even if that means a deliberate hara-kiri for malariology." He indicated that it would be no great loss because malariologists "overemphasized complexities" and the unique regional differences of the disease.

Hollow humorous references were made by other participants about the sudden eclipse of the successful old control techniques. Lewis Hackett, who had conducted several successful malaria control programs worldwide for the Rockefeller Foundation, said in a speech at the same meeting, "I am happy to be a malariologist while it is still a profession."

Brazilian malariologist Heitor P. Froes offered a poem to mark the transition from one era to the other:

> "*O Death, where is thy sting?*[5]
> Anopheles, your offspring?
> Malariologists, your job?"

Many years later malaria specialists were repeating another witticism. They said, "DDT accomplished two things. It created a super mosquito. And it eradicated malariologists." The "super mosquito" referred to the fact that mosquitoes eventually became resistant to DDT and subsequently spread disease, more successfully than ever.

Postscript

Our brief survey of the history of malaria in the United States still resisted closure. But one event fifteen years after the 4th Congress of Tropical Medicine and Malaria added the details that completed the picture.

The occasion was publication of a retrospective summary of the epidemiology of the disease in the last stages of its tenure in the U.S. South. The author was Alexander D. Langmuir, chief of the Epidemiology Branch of the U.S. Communicable Disease Center.[6]

His report marked the completion of new modernized disease surveillance and reporting units at the Center, a service that was lacking while malaria was in retreat. Langmuir's study included a review of all the old mortality and morbidity statistics during the vanishing.

He said the extensive DDT spraying program was in operation well before effective epidemiological services had been organized. "A full current evaluation of the extent of the problem had not been made."

Like so many of the doctors familiar with the unusual dynamics of the disease after the Great Depression, Langmuir knew the official statistics then were unreliable. Like those other experts, he knew that the most reliable figures were from doctors or public health officers who were reporting what they saw, not what got officially reported. In other words, doctors learned to trust what they saw and not what was reported.

When he initiated new systems for surveillance in 1947, Langmuir had noticed that the states of Mississippi, South Carolina and Texas, which reported the most cases, were using numbers that were "grossly erroneous." For their weekly malaria reports, those states listed numbers of cases instead of listing cases by names of individual patients. "Such a system encourages exaggeration," said Langmuir. Beginning in 1947, the system was changed. The figures for incidence of malaria then dropped from 17,764 to only 914 the first year. "Appraisals even among those cases revealed that only a few counted could be verified," according to Langmuir.

The epidemiologist said some time between 1935 and 1945 malaria disappeared in the United States. A slight rise in 1945 originated from World War II veterans. A steep decline followed in 1947. Then another rise in morbidity in 1951 and 1952 represented servicemen home from Korea. After that, the level stayed under 100 for the whole country, at least until the early 1970s.

Langmuir's report concluded: "The malaria story in this country should be a sobering one... Here, a disease deeply entrenched in large areas of the South disappeared within a single decade, largely, if not wholly, through natural processes rather than through planned public health measures. Even the fact of its disappearance was not appreciated until after a major control program had been in operation for several years."[7]

---

[1] It was actually the Rockefeller Sanitary Commission that started the hookworm eradication project in 1909.

[2] See 'The Great War' on pg. 139 for more details about World War I.

[3] Another important assignment was TVA's role in development of the atomic bomb used against Japan in the final days of WWII. TVA produced power in bulk for early steps in creation of the weapon.

[4] Paul Mueller was awarded the Nobel Prize for medicine in 1948 for his discovery of DDT.

[5] From: 1 Cor. 15.

[6] The Cutter Lecture on Preventive Medicine, presented at Harvard School of Public Health, Boston, May 16, 1962.

[7] See 'DDT revisited' on p. 147 for the story of DDT in other parts of the world.

PART II

The Parasite and Its Universe

It's not nice to call anyone a parasite,
A loathsome word to apply to a human being.
But the God that invented 'survival of the fittest,'
The custodian of evolution,
Surely must love parasites and need them.
Why else would she make the malaria parasite so
*   cunning?*

N.M.

Chapter 5
The Lifestyle of the Parasite

THE MALARIA STORY usually began with those daunting numbers. The headlines said several hundred million people worldwide were infected. Millions died every year, including an estimated one million young children in Africa. Actually, the malaria numbers were unreliable since the communities where the disease was most common had the least health infrastructure. The totals released to the public were estimates, and it was believed that reported cases represented about two to eight percent of the actual cases (Najera, 1992).

One source said that in the course of the history of humankind, malaria killed more people than any other single factor, including war. A statistician has calculated that malaria killed about 27 billion people throughout history, about five times the population of the world in the late 20th century (Hyde, 1990).

The story of malaria, however, was more than a damage

report. More daunting than the numbers with all the zeros trailing behind them was the rare evolutionary conditioning that allowed the parasites to defy everything the human system could muster as well as everything human beings invented to target them. Each microscopic parasite was programmed to multiply to millions within a short time in the human body. Each parasite could accommodate itself to the dangers and demands of its hosts while exploiting the hosts to satisfy its own needs. Each was a complete, single-celled animal. It consumed food, propelled itself to destinations of choice and multiplied prodigiously, by asexual and then by sexual means.

Creation of the Parasite

Modern day scientists speculated that the universe was created in an explosion some 18 billion years ago. The Earth was formed about 4.5 billion years ago and about 1.1 billion years after that, life forms emerged. Oxygen gradually replaced the original gases allowing three kingdoms of microorganisms to evolve. One of the kingdoms was the *Protista* kingdom, which was created about 1.5 billion years ago. It included the *Protozoa* phylum — or subkingdom — of animal life. Among the *Protozoa* was the *Plasmodium* genus, and that was the family group of the malaria parasites (Curtis, 1983).

Protozoa meant "first life" in Latin, placing the malaria parasites right at the roots of the tree of life. The *Protozoa* lived independently for many millions of years before evolution of the larger animals that would be their hosts and mosquitoes that would be their winged vectors. The primate-vector cycle was established around 30 million years ago. To scientists, it seemed likely that the long intimate bond between humankind and its parasites accounted for their unusual biological tolerance for each other.

Their integrated evolution was one of the most significant yet mysterious steps in the history of cells, and the pathways of molecular interactions that molded the parasitic relationship could contain far-reaching answers to basic questions about the forces of evolution (Hyde, 1990). And, of course, the evolution of the mechanisms controlling the integration of the parasites and the human hosts was a perpetual process.

The Life Cycle

The life path of the malaria parasite was a cycle. The new parasites were reproduced sexually inside a female mosquito, which then inserted the newborn creatures into the flesh of a human being or other vertebrate host. From there the parasites moved to the host's liver and then to the blood stream where they waited until time for some of them to return to the mosquito to create the next generation.

During its life cycle, the parasite moved through three distinct stages or metamorphoses, as different as an egg, a caterpillar and a butterfly. Each stage had its own shape, its own characteristics, including distinctive immunological markers expressed on its surface as antigens. At each stage in its cycle the parasite had its own work to do and path to travel.

The new malaria parasites delivered by the bite of the mosquito were called sporozoites, or pre-erythrocytes or pre-blood stage parasites. Under the microscope they looked like fragments of thread. Thousands of them entered the human tissue via the mosquito spittle, then rode on the current of human capillaries that delivered them quickly to the liver. In less than an hour, the broods were sheltered there and ready for a round of cell division.

A single sporozoite multiplied to about 30,000 to 50,000 individuals. After five to fifteen days they wormed out of the liver, assumed a new shape and a new name, merozoites. Now it was time for each to penetrate a red blood cell.

The parasites consumed hemoglobin from the blood of the host and multiplied again. After about 48 hours, each had multiplied another eight to 24 times. Then they left the ravaged blood cells in a mass explosion that made the host very sick. Typically, the victim was seized with pain, fever and chills, but the symptoms often subsided after the merozoites entered fresh red cells and settled down again to plunder, gorge and multiply. Again, parasites burst out of newly depleted blood cells, each invading still more fresh cells. Eventually there were millions of parasites in the victim's blood.

The pattern of cell destruction sometimes occurred every 48 hours in a kind of synchronization that would be reflected in a pattern of intermittent attacks of acute symptoms in the victim. In other cases, the victim was just consistently miserable. Or if the victim had suffered previous attacks of malaria he or she might respond with only mild symptoms.

The cell destruction repeated itself until the victim's immune system or medicines started to subdue the parasite or until the victim died. Before that, however, some of the parasites would undergo yet another complete metamorphosis. They became gametocytes, also called the transmission stage parasites, the critical stage in their development that prepared them for their separation into male and female forms. Then they were ready to be transported in a blood meal into a mosquito's gut where they would reproduce sexually and rejoin the cycle as new sporozoites.

The gametocyte stage occurred when the victims were very sick, such as sick babies or other individuals suffering their first episodes of what to them were new strains of the disease. Parasites that didn't reach the gametocyte stage could not reproduce to perpetuate the disease in other hosts.

The Trials of a Vector

The female mosquito was essential as a nursery and as a vector. It carried the disease from person to person, an accommodation that was reliable because mosquitoes needed blood to provide protein for their eggs. In fact the female mosquito's desire for blood was almost narcotic (BBC Online, 1998). The gametocytes rode into the mosquito's belly along with the human blood meal. In that environment the male and female forms united to create the oocysts, the egg form that allowed the creation of new sporozoites. Those moved into the mosquito's saliva and waited until the mosquito was ready for its next blood meal.

The feeding ceremony began when the mosquito landed on a victim's skin and unfurled its utensils, a package of six stylets fixed to its forehead, its proboscis. Each stylet performed a specific function. The mosquito punctured the victim's skin and prepared the wound for insertion of a tiny funnel through which the blood would travel. For the next step, the mosquito injected some of its saliva into the wound. That saliva contained an anticoagulant that prevented the incoming blood of the victim from jamming the mosquito's mouthparts. The saliva also contained something else significant: those newborn malaria parasites waiting for a new home. That was how the parasites entered the human victim.

The victim's blood flowed into the mosquito's belly, and a whole brood of young parasites flowed into the victim's flesh to start a short but eventful life of confrontations with the immune agents of the host and with medicines designed to destroy it.

The mosquitoes were marvelous disease vectors. It was hard to avoid them, and they were prodigious breeders. A female mosquito could give birth to a new generation every two weeks, from egg to egg. In five generations a single mosquito could multiply to 20 million. The rapid, massive regeneration allowed a specific population of mosquitoes to proliferate quickly in response to environmental pressures (Bates, 1949; Harrison, 1978; Tadei, 1990).

For instance, some of the mosquitoes whose environment was sprayed with DDT possessed a mutation that allowed them to neutralize the poisons effectively. Therefore, as a response to the natural pressures of survival of the fittest, they reproduced in greater numbers than the others. Over time, populations or strains emerged that were immune to insecticides.

Besides the phenomenal propensity for neutralizing threatening chemicals, some scientists believed mosquitoes could change their habits or lifestyles in a variety of ways to avoid dangers. If people they were biting put up screens, or sprayed insecticides on the bedroom walls, the mosquitoes could look elsewhere. They could go to the barn and get their blood from the farm animals. Or they could show up early at the victim's house and bite people while they sat on the porch after dinner, before they retired to the room with the insecticide on the walls.

The mosquitoes that habitually bred in a shady cove on the lake could move to the other side if developers came in with a bulldozer and ruined their privacy. Mosquitoes accustomed to life in the forest could do just fine in the rubble after the trees were cut. Mosquitoes that stayed in the forest could always feed on a variety of wild animals, whatever was handy. That's what they did before evolution brought humankind to the scene (Tadei, 1990).

Other scientists explained it differently. According to Jean E. Feagin, associate professor of pathobiology at the University of Washington, it was not changing habits that allowed mosquitoes to avoid insecticides. Rather, it was the fact that mosquito populations whose behavior made them more likely to be exposed to insecticide were killed off, leaving those with different behavior, who were there all along, to proliferate. This tended to look like a change in mosquito habits but was actually more a change in relative population density, so that mosquitoes which lived differently were now the predominant type (Feagin, 2000).

Slim Odds For Transmission

Obviously, the mathematics of malaria were colossal. Just imagine a battlefield or a riverside camp of migrating families or people in refugee camps. In settings like those, it didn't take the mosquitoes long to spread many strains of malaria over a wide area in spiraling epidemics.

After malariologists understood the dynamics of the transmission of the disease, some of them tried to create mathematical models to describe and quantify the interactions of the three: the mosquito vectors, the parasites and the human victims. That interaction, with its intricate timing, allowed the disease to flourish. One scientist in the 1950s, George Macdonald, produced formulas for those interactions, including in his calculations many factors. They included: the probable life span of the mosquitoes or of their larvae, the average number of bites a mosquito inflicted in one evening or in its lifetime, the percentage of people in an endemic community who might be gametocyte carriers, and the specific ways temperature and rainfall might effect transmission of the disease or activity of the vectors (Macdonald, 1957).

He hoped to quantify the requirements and implications of each limiting factor in the life cycle of the disease and activities of the mosquitoes so predictions might be made about the outcome of a specific epidemic or about the dimensions of the severity of an endemic presence. It was hoped that such mathematical models would be valuable in developing control strategies.

But the models didn't exactly work that way. There were just too many elusive variables in human or mosquito behavior and too many vagaries in environmental conditions where transmission took place. Because of all the vagaries and variables, it was apparent that the process of transmission of malaria from one person to another was extremely improbable, mathematically speaking.

It was becoming more and more apparent to public health workers that ongoing transmission could only take place in the presence of what appeared to be excessive numbers to beat the odds against success. The chance that any single mosquito bite would produce malaria was just too remote to reckon mathematically. Each time a mosquito completed transmission of the disease it was defying tremendous mathematical odds. Only in the presence of excessive numbers did the cycle have a chance of success.

First, not every individual *Anopheles* mosquito was a competent plasmodium carrier. There were 400 species of *Anopheles*, only 50 to 60 of them were vectors of malaria parasites (Oaks, et al., 1991).

Now, for instance, lets contemplate a competent vector looking for a blood meal. It chose a victim with exposed skin. Then assume that the intended victim had gametocytes in his or her blood. In endemic areas where most adults had some limited immunity to the disease, the odds wouldn't be great for that mosquito to pick up gametocytes in any one bite.

But, suppose the mosquito did succeed in picking up viable gametocytes in its blood meal, then succeeded in keeping them safe and finally in finding another blood source. Could that mosquito penetrate the new victim's skin deeply enough to deliver the load of new sporozoites? It didn't always work. Would the victim stay still for the necessary 15 seconds for a successful injection? Who knows?

Would the mosquito actually carry gametocytes that were mature and capable of starting the mating process for the parasites? That only happened about half the time.

When it was finished with its blood meal, could the mosquito fly away safely? They were not great flyers, especially while carrying a payload of blood many times their body weight. Some mosquitoes took in so much blood they couldn't get airborne until they had a long rest.

Another problem complicating transmission was the climate. A sudden drop in the temperature during the two weeks or so the parasites were incubating inside the mosquito could abort the process.

But assume the mosquito carrying viable gametocytes survived for two weeks or so of warm weather. Then assume the

mosquito wanted another blood meal while the next generation of new sporozoites were standing by in the saliva glands
waiting to get out, and the mosquito found someone close with
his or her sleeves rolled up. Delivery of the litter of surviving
parasites who beat the odds thus far was another long shot. According to scientists' calculations, each had just had one chance
in 20 of producing the disease. Of course, there was no chance
at all if the intended victim swatted the mosquito before it could
unfurl its stylets.

Considering all the vagaries and variables, Macdonald concluded that it was not possible to design control programs for
specific regions based on mathematical models and not possible to define just how much reduction of numbers of mosquitoes or human carriers was needed to disrupt the rate of transmission.

But his calculations convinced him of a crucial fact already
observed by malariologists working close to the problem. Given
the remote odds for transmission, one must assume there was
always a point beyond which there were not enough mosquitoes or human carriers to keep transmission going. The critical
point-of-no-return was always there, even though it was not possible to figure out precisely when that point might arrive.

Programmed to Survive

It was not necessary to eradicate mosquitoes in a community to eliminate malaria. That was noticed in the United States,
in Europe and, gradually, in other locations where the challenges were much greater. Control was possible in locations
where programs could be created to accommodate specific
needs and problems. Mosquitoes could be prevented from
breeding close to people's homes or places of work. As demonstrated in regions where land was cleared and developed, malaria could disappear without any special control programs, no
matter how many mosquitoes were around.

Macdonald also confirmed how critical the climate was in the maintenance of transmission and how transmission of malaria throughout a community was dependent on the presence of infected young children or visitors. They were the individuals who suffered the most severe cases of malaria, and thus carried the largest share of gametocytes that perpetuated the disease.

Macdonald's investigations and calculations, combined with observations of malariologists in the field, supported the realization that mosquitoes were indeed not very reliable. The disease required millions of vectors with access to gametocyte carriers to beat the odds against sustaining transmission.

The Role of the Immune System

How much of a threat, really, was the human immune system to the malaria parasite? Not much. It was believed that the human immune system was virtually incapable of preventing the infection or of clearing the disease from an infected person. The human immune system was a network of functions genetically programmed to protect the body from foreign substances, good or bad. The system worked mostly in two ways. It produced proteins called antibodies in the blood that could be activated to target a specific disease organism. The antibodies were custom-made to find, link with and destroy the enemy. That was humoral immunity.

The human immune system also included a group of white blood cells called T-cells and others, which might be activated to destroy a variety of foreign substances. Even a splinter on the finger. That nonspecific system was called cell-mediated immunity. Sometimes the two immune functions worked independently and sometimes in a partnership.

The individual suffering his or her first infection of malaria might be critically ill. If she survived, she might acquire a temporary, partial immunity to the disease that could render subsequent infections less serious. If she lived in an endemic area, she might be infected once a year or so. With each infection she would suffer less and less. People who lived all their lives in an endemic region might reach a point when they barely were aware that they were infected. But of course if she were infected by strains of malaria from other regions, the person might have a severe response to the disease, just as would a nonimmune young child.

People in endemic areas usually had what were called nonclinical infections. The immune system was activated, but the victim had no symptoms. The inactive disease was still inflicting a heavy toll on the immune system, leaving it less able to act against other infections in the neighborhood. The individual may die from measles or diarrheal disease, while acting as host to a malaria infection. People may spend almost their whole lives carrying a malaria infection that constantly made demands on their immune systems. Those folks might never know the happiness of good health, except perhaps in their old age.

Experts noted that as people in highly endemic areas aged, their immune system did not need to expend so much energy to subdue malaria infections. In fact, at the open-air markets in some endemic areas, one may notice a group of older women sitting in the shade with their basketwork in their laps, telling jokes and laughing. They'd raised their grandchildren, outlived the aggressive period of their malaria and were experiencing finally the vigor of good health.

Bonded Enemy

The malaria parasite was one enemy that the human immune system had a hard time finding and destroying. Usually the immune agents did not recognize the parasites as enemies until they had commandeered and devoured a lot of red blood cells, inflicting grave damage on the host. At least that's what it looked like to the scientists. They had several ways to explain or describe the problem.

Often the reason offered to explain the delayed reaction was the strong evolutionary bond between the human immune system and the disease organisms. In a way the two adversaries seemed to be co-dependent. The human being needed an immune mechanism to protect it from disease, and the parasite needed to learn all about that immune system and how to evade it. The "Yin and Yang" type of relationship seemed to be pulling them together and pulling them apart at the same time. Each energized the other in the evolutionary struggle for survival of the fittest.

At each of its three stages the parasite's surface proteins, or antigens, seemed to be sending different signals to the human immune system. The host's immune system recognized antigens as alarm signals about the presence of danger. Then the immune agents could target, link with, and destroy the invading disease organism. But each stage of the parasite's cycle was sending different and possibly conflicting signals. The target kept changing. The antibodies could not always be at the right place at the right time.

At each stage inside the human host, the parasite had a degree of safety. At the sporozoite stage, the malaria parasite was the most vulnerable. The antigenic markers on its surface were not as complicated as those in the other stages. But the parasite existed at the sporozoite stage only for a short period, perhaps 30 minutes. The infected person did not even feel symptoms of the disease.

The merozoites were exposed for the longest period to the threats of the immune agents and to the medicines taken by the host. That was the stage when parasites were released from the liver or from infected red cells and caused those unmistakable, devastating symptoms. That period lasted days or weeks. As might seem logical, it was the period when the parasite, particularly *P. falciparum*, displayed the most complicated and effective techniques for thwarting the human immune agents.

In addition to the shifting antigenic markers provided by its

114

three stages, the malaria parasite apparently frustrated the host's immune system in other ways. In their red blood stage the parasites, particularly *P. falciparum*, could quickly change which proteins they displayed on the surface of the infected red cells. Biologists called this aspect of the parasite's lifestyle antigenic diversity. That's different from the antigenic variety provided by stage transformations.

Scientists have identified a huge family of genes, called the *var* genes, for variability, that the parasite can mix and match to generate millions of antigenic proteins.

The parasite's obvious advantage in changing the antigens was that it prevented the human immune system from focusing its antibodies on a specific target, thus managing to stay one step ahead of the host's immune system.

Solutions Elude Specialists

Scientists didn't claim to understand all the various molecular dynamics that defined the relationship between the parasite and the human immune system. But they described in a variety of ways what seemed to be happening. The parasite appeared to have a big range of strategies for evading or immobilizing its enemies. Perhaps the parasite exaggerated its potency with superfluous antigens. This ploy would effectively delude the human immune system into expending many more antibodies than needed. The misguided immune agents themselves might then prove harmful or even fatal to the host.

There were other speculations about the activity of the merozoite. Perhaps the parasite disguised its genetic markers, creating a smokescreen effect. Then the host's immune system could not recognize the bona fide operative antigens. It appeared to scientists that the ploy thwarted an anticipated attack by antibodies. It was suggested as well that the parasite was able to mimic a component of the human immune network, thereby immobilizing it.

All those observations of course were conjecture at the time. Scientists said they really had no idea of how the human immune system functioned against malaria. But it did seem obvious that the malaria parasite knew a lot more about the human immune system than human beings knew about the parasite.

P. falciparum Specialties

In addition to a repertoire of strategies, some investigators believed that the *falciparum* parasite had the capacity to change its antigenic configuration continuously, regardless of any specific strategy or threats from human immune agents. By routinely producing sequences of new identities, the parasite was able to thrive in the absence of any effective immune response.

That was apparently what another protozoan was able to do. That other parasite was called trypanosome. It caused sleeping sickness in human beings and other diseases in cattle, and was transmitted by tsetse fly mostly in central and eastern Africa. Scientists observed that even without the presence of any threatening immune agents, the trypanosomes routinely switched the surface antigens. It was a perpetually shifting target. Later scientists could see *P. falciparum* use the same ploy.

More Enigmas

Without dispute, the malaria parasite was a master of evading the defense forces of its host without destroying it. There was a good reason. A parasite that killed its host was destroying itself in the process.

That raised an obvious question. If parasites weren't supposed to destroy their hosts, then why did falciparum malaria kill so many victims, like all those children in Africa? Ninety-five percent of all deaths due to malaria were from *P. falciparum.* That species of malaria, however, accounted for fewer than half of the cases.

One explanation of the seemingly aberrant behavior might have been the relative immaturity of *P. falciparum*. It appeared to be poorly adapted to its role as a parasite (Cook, 1989). It may not have mastered the live-and-let-live code for parasites. Some biologists have speculated that *P. falciparum* was young in evolutionary terms and less stable in its relationship with the human host than were the other species of *plasmodium*.

Some scientists believed they had evidence that *falciparum* parasites had been infecting human beings only since about 10,000 years ago. It was suggested that *P. falciparum* was very similar to the *plasmodium* parasite that infected birds and that the crossover from birds to primates could have taken place when early Hominid groups started destroying wild vegetation to plant crops (McCutchan, 1984; Rennie, 1991).

Even if it were not a model parasite, *P. falciparum* was an eminently successful organism. Enough victims obviously survived long enough to permit the mosquito vectors to pick up gametocytes and keep spreading the disease. In fact, the disease was continuing to spread even as it killed more and more of its victims. In many areas where the less deadly *P. vivax* and *P. falciparum* coexisted, the *P. falciparum* were gaining in comparison.

The *falciparum* parasite obviously was gifted, and one of the gifts was the so-called adherence factor in its blood stage. Red blood cells that were infected with *P. falciparum* adhered themselves to the inside walls of blood vessels. That protected the damaged blood cells, and the parasite within, from being swept to the spleen for destruction. The adherence was due to specific parasite-derived proteins that were exported to the surface of infected red blood cells.

Some times the infected red cells adhered to the small capillaries that fed blood to the victim's vital organs, including the brain. That apparently was at least one of the causes of cerebral malaria that killed so many young children and nonimmune travelers. There was another significant point. Those clogged capillaries might have been the reason falciparum malaria was so hard to recognize on blood slides. They were just out of sight.

Some doctors, on the other hand, did not support the theory that clogged capillaries caused all the deaths they saw from falciparum malaria. They speculated that something else might have been involved. It was suggested that perhaps large excessive accumulations of human immune agents summoned to fight the parasitic infection might have caused terminal damage to the sick person (Cannon, 1941; Sampaio, 1990).

Mysteries of the behavior of the malaria parasite kept accumulating, guaranteeing ongoing attention from some of the most accomplished scientists in the world. As always, the job of trying to understand malaria was principally a job of understanding what the parasites did to individuals and communities. That is, what kind of damage did the microbes inflict? One could speculate as well about what humankind has done to malaria. Perhaps all that medicine was helping the parasites evolve new ways of protecting themselves, making them more invincible than ever.

Behavior and Disease

By the late 1900s radical attitudes were heard about the World Health Organization and its commonly held views that could be described as paternalistic.

One criticism came from J. D. Gillett, of the Department of Medical Entomology, London School of Hygiene and Tropical Medicine, speaking at a meeting of the Royal Society of Tropical Medicine and Hygiene in 1984.

Gillett used the term 'man-made disease' to cover all communicable diseases that affect humankind as a result of his own behavior. He said, "We too often ease the passage of the vectors either by unthinkingly providing facilities for their breeding or by neglecting the simple steps that can be taken to prevent their feeding on us."

He said, "We have had nearly 100 years to try the old methods, and as far as the third world is concerned, we have failed.

Are we going to continue to put off the new phase, i.e., the study of man's active but unthinking part in the maintenance of cycles of transmission, while we forever hope for some miracle cure or preventive?"

He said, "I suggest that we must start now, not as a sideline, but as a major new activity supported by new departments in universities." He recommended that new departments first collect the data and then to plan the programs of whatever sort that are best calculated to rid us of these pestilences. He said, "During the 100 years we had to try these short cuts. But now, not only do we have the new tools, they are actually improving and becoming more suitable for our purposes as each year passes. Let us use these tools to contact the people who so often are the forgotten component in the cycles of infection we strive to prevent."

"We seem willing to pump tons of chemicals into human populations with little but local and temporary results to show for it, but reluctant to pump knowledge and understanding to the people. If profit is the driving force then perhaps it is time for a change in emphasis from chemical industry to that of the mass media. We should plan to start now even if it means reorganization on a huge scale, or be judged on why we failed to act."

Speaking about malaria, he said, "It seems incomprehensible that we should spend so much time, money and effort studying the behavior of the parasite and the invertebrate host and neglect almost entirely the third component that so often makes these many and varied cycles of transmission important, namely the behavior of man."

He added, "Immunology and the hope of vaccination against malaria may have delayed the implementation of this new approach, i.e. the study of the effects of man's behavior in the transmission of the disease."

Gillett also mentioned the bubonic plague that "mysteriously" disappeared from Uganda in the early 1940s. Uganda, in those days flourished financially mainly because of two introduced cash crops: coffee and cotton, both of which brought great wealth to the country.

He said, "The disappearance of plague from Uganda coincided with the introduction of antibiotics and DDT but probably had nothing to do with either, just as the virtual disappearance of malaria from the U.S.A. in the 1950s (which stood at 4 million cases per year in the 1930s) had little, if anything to do with the new antimalarials and DDT."

Gillett continued, "I well remember L. W. Hackett emphasizing this point when I was studying epidemiology at Berkeley in 1955. In U.S.A, as in Western Europe, changes in the ways of man were probably involved. Perhaps some of us should be making a special study of the factors involved in bringing these great recessions with as much energy as we bring to the study of the factors responsible for the establishment of endemic and epidemic conditions."

Chapter 6
World History

A S THE READER knew by now, the family of malaria parasites was almost as old as life on Earth. For millions and millions of years, new animals evolved, including ancestors of humankind, of *Plasmodium* and of mosquitoes. After the three were joined in a cycle, the malaria parasite had everything it needed to participate as a major force in the course of human history.

Experts believed that Africa, called the "cradle of humankind," could also be called the "cradle of malaria." The receding glaciers of the Pleistocene had rendered parts of Africa a lush and safe environment of enclosed arboreal canopies, permitting parasitic organisms to move among various animals, testing relationships.

As the glaciers to the north receded for the last time, African forests began to thin out and dehydrate, a process that continued at least into the 21st century. Many of the larger species, including the prehominid apes, lost their trees in the climate change and had to adapt to life on the ground. They learned to balance on two feet, live in groups, search for food and use tools. Gradually some of the hominids must have extended their territories to satisfy their needs. They found neighbors to consolidate their communities and identified enemies they would feel obliged to battle in defense of their territory. Humankind evolved for millions of years during that transition, first as *Homo habilis*, next as *Homo erectus*, then finally as *Homo sapiens*. That was modern humankind. Scientists believed *Homo* was malarious before it was *sapiens*.

Family Pictures

It was easy for the modern day armchair scientist to imagine the setting. Popular books, magazines and museum displays offered appealing artistic representations of the life of early man. Bones and footprints discovered by the famous Leaky family and others in or near the Olduvai Gorge in Tanzania tantalized scientists and the general public all over the world. Ancient footprints as old as 3.6 million years and other relics inspired visions of ape-like families with scowling faces walking single file across the savanna, mountains smoking in the background (Agnew, et al., 1998).

As groups from different regions mingled, their strains of parasites got to mingle as well. Everyone was exposed to new species and strains of *Plasmodium* for which they had no immunity. There have been speculations that that might have been how the disease of malaria got started.

Paleohistorians believed that prehistoric human groups then spread out over many thousands of years in several directions, eventually populating much of the globe's dry land. Experts speculated that, during their evolution, humankind and other animals had developed the spleen to accommodate the debris of all the red blood cells destroyed by their fellow travelers, the malaria parasites. In fact, from Hippocrates times to the present, an enlarged spleen signaled a malaria infection to doctors. At a much later date the early people moved across the thick shoulders of the African continent, presumably contributing to a trail of sickle cell. That was the defective red blood cell that rendered some African people at least partially immune to malaria. The sickle cell shielded red blood cells from penetration by the malaria parasite (Durham, 1991, p.125). It was believed the misshapen cell was selected genetically in response to the advantage it gave to humankind over malaria. Scientists believed that other red blood defects emerged in early humankind as well, but those others were not so clearly understood.

Besides the western trek, historians determined that early African people must have traveled in other directions, southward and also northward down the Nile. The north route linked people close and far. Those included the ancient Egyptians, whose remains were found in tombs. From Egypt, Africans linked as well with the early trade routes leading east out to Mesopotamia and extending as far as India and China where people perfected healing techniques, still administered successfully in modern times to millions of patients (Ackerknecht, 1992).

Ancient Greece

In their push north to the underbelly of Europe, the last glaciers of the *Pleistocene*, or Ice Age, uncovered the rocky peninsula and submerged islands of Greece. The area warmed to temperatures of modern times, and in the wake of the ice came a variety of animals attracted by the improved conditions. The animals provided blood meals needed for *P. falciparum*-bearing mosquitoes that thrived in the new moderate climate.

When humankind appeared, they disrupted the environment, cutting down trees to make their own space. It was typical of pioneers everywhere. The evicted animals moved deeper into the wilderness for food and privacy. Mosquitoes then took their blood meals from the human beings and used the new litters of advancing civilization to breed in.

Historians had several tools for assigning dates to the transformation of Greece, including the warming, the arrival of humankind, the new agriculture and the emergence of malaria. Clues were found in sediment from extinct lakebeds left dry by glacial movements. More clues were found in bones, in literature and in art objects.

The sediment contained the most valuable information for fixing the dates for geological changes and for the arrival of people in the lush, reclaimed land. It was calculated that people arrived in Greece in 8300 BC (Grmek, 1991).

Early Greek literature was drawn on to estimate the arrival of human malaria there. Many experts cited the prodigious analyses of William Henry Samuel Jones (1876–1963), a leading scholar in Greek history and literature. Jones maintained that malaria must have arrived in Greece after 500 BC, during the classical period. He concluded the disease raged from the Hellenistic period until the 20th century. He based his ideas in part on specific works of Homer, Hippocrates and others, and on the record of intermittent wars and social upheaval of the period. By that time, the Greeks, Spartans and some of their neighbors were developing a cultural ethos of war and battle heroism.

A passage from Book XXII of Homer's *Iliad,* the epic history of the Trojan War written in the 8th century BC, was frequently cited. Homer described the berserk battle rage of Achilles as he attacked his enemies, and the poet compared it to the common outbreaks of deadly fevers that reached their peak each year in the fall. Homer identified the season with the star Sirius, "Orion's Dog," which was most prominent in the autumn sky.

The aged Priam was the first of all whose eyes saw him
As he swept across the flat land in full shining, like that star
Which comes on in the autumn and whose conspicuous
    brightness

Far outshines the stars that are numbered in the night's dark-
ening,
The star they give the name of Orion's Dog, which is the brightest
Among the stars, and yet is wrought as a sign of evil
And brings on the great fever for unfortunate mortals.

(Translation by Lattimore)

The most precise early descriptions of malaria came from
Hippocrates. He traveled throughout the region and described
vividly the effects and ecology of the disease, leaving the im-
pression with some historians that he was describing something
new. But what he saw was apparently very old.

CLASSIFICATION OF TYPES OF MALARIA TRANSMISSION IN DIFFERENT REGIONS

Holoendemic: Intense year-round malaria transmission,
where the population's level of immunity is high, particularly among adults.

Hyperendemic: Seasonal transmission of malaria, where the
population's level of immunity does not confer adequate
protection from disease for all age groups.

Mesoendemic: Some malaria transmission, although occa-
sional epidemics constitute a heavy public health burden due to low levels of immunity.

Hypoendemic: Limited malaria transmission, where the
population has little or no immunity to the parasite.

(Source: *Malaria, Obstacles and Opportunities,* Institute of Medicine,
1991)

Evidence and Theory

Modern studies, including studies in paleopathology, have
drawn circumstantial evidence that malaria actually arrived in
Greece with the earliest human settlements in 8300 BC. That

deduction was founded on the expanding awareness among scientists of the record of falciparum malaria's initial devastating confrontations with inexperienced communities. The scientists suggested the malaria attacks alluded to by writers of the Hellenistic Era were recrudescences of the first hyperendemics.[1] There apparently were three or four large waves of falciparum malaria across the face of Greece before the beginning of the Roman period.

Scientists of the 20th century also were learning more about a hereditary anemia that damaged bone marrow of its victims causing several defects, including grotesque configurations of their cranial structure. Some of the facial bones were enlarged and some were hollowed out, creating a smashed-in appearance.

The disease was popularly called thalassemia and was known scientifically as cranial porotic hyperostosis. Scientists found similarities among thalassemia and other hereditary human anemias that provided some immunity to malaria. The connection became clear as investigations showed that the modern-day presence of the thalassemia trait was identified with areas of Greece and its neighbors. Those areas also had historic records of violent malaria.

Investigators concluded that somehow ancient hyperendemics of malaria in Greece must have selected for that genetic defect in following generations. But of course a long time lag must have separated the initial assault and the later emergence of the subsequent defect. Many paleopathologists and other scientists have examined bones of victims, as well as some of the few victims in modern times who still carried the ancient traits. Apparently there was no evidence to date the earliest appearance of the defect (Grmek, 1991).

The dormant gene or trait for the disease was detected in routine blood tests of children and adults in 1948–1955 in widely separated areas. The trait was most commonly seen in Greece and elsewhere in the eastern Mediterranean.

The thalassemia genetic marker also was detected in routine

tests on hospital patients and armed service personnel. Studies showed that some of the locations in Greece and surrounding areas where the gene appeared most frequently were known to be regions with a history of severe malaria, in addition to a history of sickle cell disease or other hereditary anemias linked with malaria.

In modern times in the eastern Mediterranean, it was still possible to see an individual with the full-blown thalassemia. Some living people with the full stigmata of the disease have been reported also among isolated tribal people in the forests of Southeast Asia (Sharma and Kondrashin, 1991).

A Visit To the Louvre

One medical historian who researched evidence on thalassemia was surprised by a collection of terra cotta figurines he saw at the Louvre Museum in Paris. He was Mirko D. Grmek, Director of Studies at L'Ecole Pratique des Hautes Etudes at the Sorbonne and president of the International Academy of the History of Science from 1981 to 1985.

The figurines were from the Hellenistic era, depicting children with the protruding facial bones and crushed noses typical of thalassemia. Seven figurines came from Smyrna. One was found at Troy. Both were cities of the ancient Greek world. Grmek wrote that he looked at several other specimens of Smyrnean sculpture in the collection, which proved to him that the artists' goal was to depict an actual pathological state, "not an imaginative search for the 'grotesque'" (Grmek, 1991).

The figurines, of course, did not prove that violent early attacks of falciparum malaria against earlier Greek inhabitants were responsible for thalassemia in the Hellenistic period. But they did seem to offer support for the argument that those malaria outbreaks described by Homer, Hippocrates and others were not part of the first wave of falciparum malaria in Greece. Meanwhile, scientists were finding indications that hyperendemics must have struck Greece three times before malaria reached its apogee about the time Rome seized dominance of the region in 31 BC.

Grmek was convinced of the need for more comprehensive research to address issues raised by the multiple enigmas of thalassemia. He said investigators needed "to consider the plurality of hematozoic parasites,[2] their biological history and that of their vectors, human migrations, archaeological data and finally, recent discoveries of paleoclimatology and physics of the planet" *(Ibid.)*.

Hippocrates

Western historians have been unified about the validity of Hippocrates. His practice, research and writing made him a monument to the art of medicine, and he set professional and ethical standards that were a measure of quality for centuries to come.

Hippocrates introduced a biographical approach to diagnosing and treating illness: talking to his patients at great length about their symptoms, their personal history, the history of their families, their living conditions, and their social and physical environment. He described malaria with particular precision. He recorded the first correlation in the West between the proximity to bodies of water and the stricken communities. He also offered an accurate anatomy of the disease's symptoms: enlarged spleens, intermittent fevers and violent chills.

While Hippocrates successfully charted the characteristics of malaria, he did not address its true etiology. His view of illness was largely guided by the philosophy of Empedocles, who held that the entire universe or macrocosm, including the microcosm of the human body, was made of four elements or "humors." Those were water, air, fire and earth (Ackerknecht, 1992). For the healthy individual, according to that popular theory, the four elements were perfectly balanced. Illness was caused when the natural balance had been disrupted. Modern scholars believed that the doctrine, which dominated medical thinking in the Western world for many centuries, originated in India and came to Greece via Egypt. The eclectic cultural borrowing would have been characteristic of ancient Greece, which soaked up the knowledge and traditions from many different regions of the ancient world like a giant sponge. Many historians believed that one explanation of Greece's apparent intellectual success was that the people knew when and what to borrow from other cultures. One clearly original contribution, however, of the ancient Greeks to the world in general and to medical science in particular was the passion for thorough compilation and categorization of knowledge. Hippocrates' notes and lectures, compiled by Alexandrian scholars in the third century BC, filled 72 volumes and covered virtually all the medical information known to the ancient world (Grmek, 1991).

One historian said: "Greek medicine was a 'resurrection' of the scientific tradition of Egypt and the Near East. Homer's *Iliad* credited Egypt as the place where Greek drugs originated. Several scientific observations from the famous *Edwin Smith* and *Ebers Papyri*[3] were repeated twelve centuries later in the *Corpus Hippocraticum*" (Inglis, 1965).

Downfall of the Empire

Historians speculated about the possibility that malaria caused the downfall of ancient Greek culture (Grmek, 1991). The conclusion usually was yes, but with qualifications. There were certainly other causes for the disarray that led to the collapse of Greece. The empire was weakened by the growth and excesses of the upper classes. The suppression of slaves, workers and traders led to political unrest. The centralized powers were unable to control isolated rural communities, and invasions by "barbarians" from central Europe threatened the stability of the empire (Langer, 1980).

When the Roman Empire gained dominance of the eastern Mediterranean region, it inherited ancient Greek medical traditions but squandered the legacy, according to historians. The Hippocratic medical traditions were dissipated by the Roman emphasis on religion, the supernatural and superstition. Rome did, however, set examples for modern public health and sanitation. Three Roman authors first proclaimed the theory that small animals and insects emerging from swamps were responsible for the ubiquitous fevers in the region. That theory inspired the sewage systems of the sixth century BC. Later, aqueducts were constructed to supply portions of the empire with fresh water. The water works, however, did not reach far enough to serve a large area, and most of the population continued to suffer badly from malaria and other diseases. Nevertheless, Roman water systems became models for public health protection in many countries throughout history.

Periodic wars and sickness handicapped Rome as it extended its territorial reaches far beyond its capacity to administer new regions. The eventual collapse of agriculture added to the misery, and the Romans were not able to defend themselves from northern invaders. Did malaria contribute to the fall of Rome? As with the case of the ancient Greek Empire, historians have answered this question equivocally. It was possible that malaria actually postponed the inevitable collapse of Rome. There was so much malaria along the empire's northern borders that invading forces often had to stop for long periods to recover from the disease or to wait for new troops to replace them. Malaria, of course, wasn't the only disease incapacitating the citizenry. Regions with inadequate housing or plumbing and shifting populations were magnets for many infectious diseases.

The Dark Times

As the Roman Empire disintegrated, much of Europe fell into what has been called the "Dark Ages," and the long period of chaos following Rome's collapse was indeed dark in many ways. Wars were persistent, and military victories were only temporarily decisive. The agricultural infrastructure, including the famous roads Rome built throughout much of southern Europe, was in ruins. Disease was rampant. But according to historians, the sick were neglected or simply left to die. Epidemics, including the plague, typhus, dysentery, scarlet fever, measles, cholera and malaria, swept back and forth across the ruined lands of the former empires. Historians of medicine were convinced that malaria was rampant, but there were no systems for diagnosis or record keeping. And malaria was probably not as visible or fatally aggressive as were other diseases.

Ancient Greek science, philosophy and medicine had largely disappeared from Europe in the Dark Ages. Then, Arab and North African scholars reintroduced many of those crucially important traditions to Europe in the course of the Muslim colonization of the Iberian Peninsula, starting in the early eleventh century. The works of Hippocrates were revived by Arab scholars and doctors, who developed an advanced medical theory and practice. Public sanitation and extensive waterworks not seen in Europe since the height of the Roman Empire were reintroduced. Almost simultaneously, scholars of the Ottoman Empire were reviving and developing many aspects of ancient Greek philosophy and science, including the Hippocratic traditions. Those cultural influences from the Muslim south and east contributed in many ways to the development of the European renaissance during the thirteenth century and to the foundations of the European university system, which became the bedrock of modern Western medicine.

From the late middle ages through the early modern period, malaria continued to ravage the European continent. That was when the term itself was coined. "Malaria," the Italian expression for "bad air," referred to the prevalent notion that the fevers, chills, enlarged spleens and deaths were caused by noxious vapors rising from swamps and stagnant pools of water. The old word "ague" gradually lost its currency.

Rich and powerful people throughout Europe were no more

immune to the depredations of "the ague" than were the common folk. More notable victims of the disease included Alexander the Great, St. Augustine (first Archbishop of Canterbury), King James I, King Charles II, Cardinal Wolsey and Oliver Cromwell (Cook, 1990). Malaria also disrupted the politics of the Vatican. Pope Sixtus V died of the disease, as did his successor, Pope Urban VII. Many delegates were fatally infected on their way to the Vatican conclave in 1623. Eight cardinals of the Holy Roman Church and 30 of their secretaries died of the disease during the same period, and many more became ill (Covell, 1967; Celli, 1933).

New Compassion

Beginning in the seventeenth century, more effective and compassionate attention was directed toward healing the citizenry of a wide variety of ailments. For a long period, the standard cures for just about every internal ailment had been lancing, purging, bleeding and cautery. Eventually, new discoveries about germs and modes of contagion lay the foundations for modern practice, and a new wave of enlightened doctors began to lead the profession.

One of them was Thomas Sydenham (1624–1689), who was called the "English Hippocrates." Among his contributions to modern medicine were the scientific classification of various conditions, illnesses, and their respective treatments, and also the systematic and precise recording of dosage levels of prescription medications. In addition he recorded precise measurements of patient outcomes.

Sydenham "rationalized" medicine, rejecting the old practice of polypharmacy or the use of a variety of drugs without regard for the specific symptoms of the patient. Sydenham rejected, as well, excessive and intrusive methods of bloodletting and cautery. Sydenham based his theories on scientific experimentation, and paid special attention to common ailments, including malarial fevers, and to the medical details of the personal hygiene and surroundings of a patient. He had a reputation as a compassionate, gentle and modest man, never taking credit for a patient's recovery. He praised instead the patient's own resilience and God's life-creating powers. In that way, he helped to set the medical standards for his generation and to lay the foundations of modern medical ethics (Bruce-Chwatt, 1980).

Quinine

In 1633, reports spread from Barcelona about a "new" medicine from Peru, a powder made from the bark of "fever trees" in the province of Luja. The Augustan missionary who reported the discovery claimed that the powder cured malaria. He said, "One hears of its miraculous effects in Lima" (Bruce-Chwatt, 1988). Physicians and pharmacologists moved fast. Within 20 years of the first report, Sydenham and his colleagues in Britain were testing, prescribing and administering the drug with good results. In 1672, an apprentice apothecary used the bark powder to cure King Charles II of "the resistant ague." The reward was knighthood and the King's protection from "the molestations and disturbance" of the Royal College of Physicians (*Ibid.*). One could only guess what those physicians wanted to do to the apothecary.

Quinine was a breakthrough in European medicine as well as a breakthrough for Latin American herbal cures. While some doctors approached a rational and scientific medical practice, many practitioners still relied on old theories such as the "four humors" and on old-style brutal treatment techniques. But with the fever bark tree, people had a realistic expectation of a reliable, single medicine that targeted a specific disease, perhaps the most destructive disease of its time.

Botanical exploration parties from several European countries and adventurers headed to the South American jungles to look for the "fever trees." The trees came to be called cinchona, loosely named for the first wife of the Viceroy of Peru. International controversies arose about the exploitation of the trees and about the trade itself. Apparently there were wide discrepancies in the medicinal value of the trees' various strains, and some were easier than others to export, transplant and harvest.

Producing the medicine from the bark was difficult. The alkaloids that brought such fast relief were mixed in many different and sometimes ineffective or dangerous ways. In 1820, almost 200 years after cinchona's introduction to Europe, two French chemists created a reliable formula for preparing the drug, based on its principle alkaloid, quinine.

It would be hard to exaggerate the public enthusiasm for the product. The medicine was fast acting and reliable. In fact, quinine was so reliable that it soon became popular as a diagnostic tool. A doctor would first treat a terrible fever with quinine. If the patient's condition did not improve, the doctor would know that it was not malaria they were looking at. Then he would proceed to another possible diagnosis.

The inevitable race to control production of the trees was marked by confusion and contention, with botanists and chemists from several European countries competing for domination of the industry. The keenest competition was between England and the Netherlands, both having colonies in Asia with a good climate, fertile land for the trees and cheap labor for the plantations.

But several early attempts to start new stands of trees met with failure. The Netherlands, which reportedly did the best homework, finally was able to assemble what turned out to be the most reliable strains of tree. The Netherlands established profitable cinchona plantations in Indonesia, which dominated the market until well into the twentieth century (Bruce-Chwat, 1988).

Beginning in the early 1800s in the western world, developments and attitudes were changing fast. Discoveries and advances in medical science and the development of eastern practices led to the invention of the stethoscope, the use of the microscope for diagnosis, the popularization of autopsies for medical analysis, the use of ether for operations, the development of drainage networks and safe sewage systems to prevent epidemics, sterilization of open wounds, the realization that every disease had a microscopic origin and the discovery of X-rays. In other developments, Pasteur disproved the theory of the spontaneous generation of disease organisms, and epidemiologists John Snow and William Budd demonstrated that disease organisms were waterborne.

Bills of Mortality

Among some leaders in Europe, a need was recognized for collaboration on health issues. The First International Medical Congress met in Paris in 1867 to allow health care providers and leaders to open a cross-border dialogue for the exchange of ideas on disease prevention, control and treatment of the principal infections. Several meetings were held. No specific continent-wide disease-control projects were undertaken, but the idea survived. Some historians have suggested the possibility of a lack of harmony among the group. Giving up separate national priorities could be difficult at first. One issue may have involved personal or national status. Italy, for instance, was known to be home to some of the most famous and competitive malaria specialists on the continent, and home also to some of the most devastating malaria epidemics in history. Unlike its neighbors, Italy supported total reliance on quinine for protecting its population. Effective international collaboration was yet to come.

Europe continued to be a very unhealthy place. Besides the disease toll exacted by intermittent warfare, the emerging Industrial Revolution was igniting new disease, or old disease in new places. Poor families from rural areas were migrating to the cities, where the adults and their children could get jobs in the new factories. Much of the movement was the result of land enclosures by large landowners and the consequent breakdown of traditional feudal systems.

Typically, the congested cities lacked adequate housing, sanitation and fresh food. The results were inevitable. Diseases that had been sweeping the land moved into the cities, and devastating epidemics erupted. They included smallpox, dysentery, typhus and malaria.

The most critical disease in London then was cholera. Historians said a point was reached when the uncontrollable urban cholera epidemics threatened the political stability of Britain's government. In 1875, London passed a comprehensive public health act providing that sewage systems, pure water and other hallmarks of disease prevention and control were finally regarded as the responsibility of the state (Learmonth, 1988).

Another example of forceful public health reform was in Russia. Johanna Peter Franck (1745–1821,) physician to Czar Alexander I, declared that the Russian State was responsible for citizens' health. He issued a treatise on public health covering, among other topics, sewage, water supply and school hygiene. In addition, France had gained a reputation for its leadership in public health development.

Some historians called the emerging period the Age of Preventive Medicine. Meanwhile, several writers were rallying public opinion to recognize the poor state of sanitation and health, mainly in the cities. The prominent lawyer Sir Edwin Chadwick released a report in 1842 exposing the dangerous health conditions of the laboring classes. He used statistical evidence from Dr. William Farr, who three years previously published detailed reports on causes of death in England.

Malaria, which had devastated much of Europe and the United States in earlier times, was receding naturally. A big boost for malaria control was the new knowledge about successful projects in the U.S. South for reducing transmission of the disease, without the benefit of special control or treatment strategies. Sanitation engineers were learning more about the techniques perfected in parts of the U.S. South including the Tennessee Valley Authority project, and about the Cuba and Panama control projects. Sanitation engineers could adapt the new lessons from entomologists about the lifestyle and breeding habits of the various anophelines. Another reality should not be ignored. Prosperity always was the best weapon against malaria.[4]

In Western countries, life expectancy rose from 40 years in 1850 to 70 years in 1950. One commentator of the time said the rise was due more to preventive than to curative medicine. He was Oliver Wendell Holmes (1809–1894), famous American writer, physician and jurist. He was an outspoken champion of the public health reform, writing that "the bills of mortality are more affected by drainage than by this or that method of medical practices."

Mosquito Finally Convicted

Just as quinine had revolutionized the treatment of malaria, two discoveries by European army doctors revolutionized the science of the disease. In 1880, Alphonse Laveran, a French pathologist and army physician stationed in Algeria, discovered the parasite of human malaria. Then, in 1897 a British army doctor stationed in India, Ronald Ross, made the discovery that mosquitoes transmitted malaria and opened doors for effective prevention strategies that would save an uncountable number of lives throughout the world.

Then, Ross was among the first of several specialists who set out to create rational malaria-control projects in the tropics.

Mosquitoes In the Colonies

Europe accelerated its long preoccupation with empire building. England, France, Spain, the Netherlands, Germany, Portugal and Italy were establishing and expanding colonies in the tropics. Between 1870 and 1900, the United States and European powers added almost 120 million people and 10 million square miles to their empires. Almost all of it was malarious. In India in an ordinary year, 100 million people were sick with malaria, and 1 million died.

The Ross Institute of Tropical Hygiene became affiliated with the London School of Hygiene and Tropical Medicine, which undertook several control projects. Soon tropical plantations, mines, shipping companies, slave trade, and poppy fields were creating fortunes for the absentee owners. Consequently, there was money to spare for malaria control, using strategies designed by scientists from the home country. France, Italy and the Netherlands chose medications as the main instrument for malaria control in their colonies. In territories ruled by British and the U.S., vector control was the strategy of choice (Herms, et al., 1940).

Challenge For the New Doctor

One of the earliest big projects after Ross's discovery about mosquito vectors was at a British colony in Southeast Asia, the Federated Malay States, later called Malaya, and then Malaysia. A newly graduated British naval doctor, Malcolm Watson, arrived there in 1901 for his first overseas assignment as district surgeon of Klang district, south of Kuala Lumpur. His territory was a low coastal plateau planted in rubber and surrounded by marshes and mangrove swamps. Tidal waters and heavy rains intermittently inundated the area. Malaria was rampant.

The colonial administrators had ordered new labor from Ceylon. The workers, imported originally from China, were nonimmune to the strains of the disease in their new home and, quinine was not effective as a treatment or prevention (Herms et. al, 1940). Adding to the workers' misery was the fact that the mosquitoes of Southeast Asia were particularly aggressive and, as Watson learned, unpredictable.

The new medical officer constructed sluices, rechanneled streams and installed locks to permit tidal water to flow in and out. The purposes were to irrigate crops, drain standing water and flush out areas inhabited by larvae. Watson was learning and improvising all the way. He was also familiarizing himself with the several local species of mosquito vectors and their characteristics, especially their breeding and biting preferences. That way he could direct his control methods to target vectors delivering the most trouble.

It was called "species sanitation," and Watson was considered a pioneer in the art. But a surprising problem developed that was not easy to understand. He found that some species of mosquito had double lives: one behavior pattern for the hills and another for the lowlands, or different behaviors in the monsoons and dry seasons. Effective control strategies were slow in coming. It took Watson about 16 years to finish the job. He later shared his new techniques at control projects in other English colonies.

Meanwhile, back in Europe, continued intermittent warfare among kingdoms, republics and lesser jurisdictions continued to exact a heavy toll in terms of malaria and other diseases. The regional conflicts, national rivalries and antagonisms continued to gain momentum, and by the turn of the century a full-scale war erupted, then known as the Great War.

The Great War

World War I (1914–1918), which was called the Great War until a bigger one came along, was different from the many previous wars that had scarred Europe throughout its history. The war eventually involved more than 16 countries in two alliances. But it accomplished next to nothing politically in terms of shoring up foundations for lasting peace. As one historian pointed out, "a process of 50 years had gone to make Europe flammable, and a few days were enough to detonate it" (Britannica, 1965). Twenty-one years after the war ended with the Versailles treaty, Europe was suffering through the second installment.

The First World War caught fire on June 28, 1914, with the assassination of the Archduke Francis Ferdinand in Sarajevo. The result was Germany's declaration of war on France. Other nations quickly lined up to join in the fray.

As in other wars, malaria was the hidden enemy aimed at both sides. The war was fought on many fronts. The Macedonia campaign on the southern front has been cited frequently over the years for its extreme futility. Opposing troops there were immobilized for three years by malaria.

From 1916 to 1918, an average of 124,000 British troops were engaged in battle, and 162,152 hospital admissions were attributed to malaria. An estimated 2 million "man days" were lost to the disease in 1918 alone. Obviously, some troops got malaria over and over again, or kept getting sick from repeated episodes of the same infection. Men and boys evacuated for malaria were replaced by other soldiers, who in turn would become sick themselves. Combatants from other countries were also sidelined by the disease. In the heat of the fighting, one French commanding general at Macedonia was ordered to attack. He telegraphed a terse reply back to central command: "Regret that my Army is in hospital with malaria" (Ognibene and Barrett, 1982).

The Macedonia campaign confirmed that quinine alone was not successful in preventing or curing the disease and that military and civilian doctors had to re-educate themselves about malaria's ferocity (Barber, 1929). Doctors already realized that quinine, the perennial battlefield choice, just didn't work to suppress the disease or prevent it. In previous war or peacetime outbreaks, the medicine at least suppressed the disease, slowing it down long enough for the combatants to get on their feet and function satisfactorily until the next episode. In World War I, however, doctors realized that the disease was actually developing resistance to quinine. It was not always easy to get up and function again (Tigertt, 1966).

Environmental Casualties

The war left Europe in shambles. It precipitated a breakdown in administration, transportation, distribution of medical supplies and housing construction. The war also allowed unprecedented mingling of nonimmune people with people in advanced stages of malaria. Those were the sick people who carried the infectious gametocytes.

Peacetime was just about as bad as wartime in terms of malaria transmission. Combatants returned home to farms that had been systematically turned into battlefields. An American malariologist observed that "the killing or removal of livestock and the destruction of stables may tend to force zoophilic[5] species to feed more often on man. In addition, the stabling of military animals in the middle of a village may attract unusual numbers of a vector species" (Russell, 1952).

Russia suffered the most. The epidemic there of 1922 took place as a result of World War I. It was considered the largest European epidemic of modern times, extending as far north as the Arctic Circle and causing millions of deaths (Ognibene and Barrett, 1982). Some people say that the unusually warm temperatures of that year may have greatly contributed to the epidemic.

Two Strategies

The subsequent war on malaria was fought on two fronts, one favoring environmental manipulations to minimize contact between disease vectors and potential victims. The other front was a search for new medicines or chemical products to replace quinine. The two strategies were on diverging tracks.

The Rockefeller Foundation emphasized the first track. By 1924, it had established a network of research institutions in 26 countries. Malariologists staffed each bureau and traveled to various projects. Rockefeller scientists conducted projects from start to finish or merely helped local scientists identify specific malaria trouble spots and demonstrate ways to seek corrections. It was the first international program designed to combat a single disease and the first program with enough money and expertise to identify rationally what worked and what didn't.

One of the projects Rockefeller scientists masterminded was in Brazil. It began in 1932 as a yellow fever control project. That disease, carried by *Aedes aegypti* mosquitoes, was never as difficult as malaria to control. As soon as the job was done, a Rockefeller field entomologist in Brazil spotted an *Anopheles gambiae* a long way from home. That was bad news. The *An. gambiae*, a large, long-lived, and prolific malaria vector, had been confined to Africa, stowing away sometimes on boats down the Nile and stopping in Sudan. Sometimes the mosquitoes crossed the border into Suez, where health authorities usually could control them.

The mosquito experts working in Brazil figured the *An. gambiae* there had stowed away to Natal on a ship from West Africa. Apparently the invaders then transferred to a slow boat or truck, making frequent stops along the coastal meadows to take a blood meal or lay a batch of eggs. The Rockefeller scientists, led by Fred Soper in collaboration with Brazilian government staff, stalked the mosquito up the coast. They focused on the periphery of mosquito colonies, clearing breeding sites with Paris Green or pyrethrum. Under pressure, large colonies broke up and shrank until malaria was no longer sustainable. It took years, but it worked.

Many residents had fled for the cities. The human toll was huge. In 1938, 100,000 people got malaria; 20,000 died. In 1939, 185,572 were infected. In 1940, the number was 6,124. By the mid-1940s, the *An. gambiae* were gone. Historians gave credit for the victory mainly to Soper's strategy of moving slowly against one well-defined colony at a time. In addition, Soper was able to analyze the mosquitoes' behavior and anticipate their moves. Historians said later that the project proved it was possible to dislocate a species of mosquito from a specific area with the right information, materials and patience.

League of Nations

The year the Rockefeller team began its coordinated work in Europe, 1924, was the year that the League of Nations established its Malaria Commission.[6] Its principal functions were to conduct inspection tours within Europe and to report the findings. The commission's first reports seemed to reflect the findings of pioneer malariologists in the U.S. South. The analyses sounded pessimistic to some people first, but later were regarded as logical and helpful. Examples:

"The history of special antimalarial campaigns is chiefly a record of exaggerated expectations followed sooner or later by disappointments and abandonment of work."
1927. Special report, Malaria Commission of the League of Nations.

"What is required is that each medical officer of health should be the malaria officer for the district he controls. It may take years to collect data, but each individual observation, if accurate, is of the greatest value. The aggregate of data slowly and steadily recorded will in time form the basis on which sound economical work can be established."
From a League of Nations memorandum of antimalarial measures in the Punjab, India.

A growing number of malaria specialists could not accept a go-slow strategy. They were certain a universal solution, a winning medicine or insecticide, was just around the corner. The faith in the larvicide Paris Green and the insecticide pyrethrum gained in popularity for a while. Paris Green , however, started to lose favor. The reasons offered were similar to the reasons that TVA managers in the U.S. rejected Paris Green. It was too expensive for most people in malarious regions. And it was considered hazardous to the environment. The formula included arsenic. Pyrethrum used alone or with other insecticides was popular and effective until it was eclipsed by DDT in the 1940s. Later, after DDT was discredited, pyrethrum regained popularity, both for indoor and agricultural spraying.

Search For Better Medicines

The shocking malaria epidemics in postwar Europe and the apparent failure of quinine to control the disease stimulated pharmaceutical companies everywhere to try to create new medicines. The early focus was a search for synthetic versions of the old medicine quinine. Experiments with artificial antimalarials were based on a class of compounds known as 4-amino quinolines, the chemical composition of quinine. One product that attracted immediate attention was resochin, developed in 1934 by a German pharmaceutical company. A few years later it was modified and produced as sontochin.

In 1943, U.S. scientists acquired the formula and technology for producing sontochin when Tunis was liberated from the Germans. Its composition was modified again slightly and finally issued under still another name, chloroquine. No one would argue that the final product was not worth the effort.

The new synthetic drug caused a sensation in the rarefied world of tropical medicine — though nothing, of course, like the furor caused by its organic counterpart 300 years earlier. Chloroquine soon became the drug of choice for malaria treatment everywhere. It cured malaria and prevented the disease when taken as prophylaxis. In addition, it was cheap and easily tolerated, even by children and pregnant women.

Post World War II

World War II was different from World War I in several ways and also the same.[7] In the First World War, U.S. troops were barely used, but U.S. factories supplied essential war materials. In World

War II, weaponry on all fronts was much more modern and deadly, and the toll of U.S. participants killed in action tremendous, yet small in comparison with the German and Russian casualties. For many years after peace was signed the major foreign policy goal everywhere was to prevent a number three.

Malaria was critically destructive in both wars. But in World War II, military doctors had access to new weapons: DDT and chloroquine. They also had access to laboratories experimenting with alternative drugs.

Even by 1945, however, specialists had noted that falciparum malaria had the capacity to resist at least some of the new compounds (Tigertt, 1972).

Drug Resistance

By the late 1950s, scientists in India and in the U.S. saw indications that the malaria parasite was acquiring resistance to chloroquine. In addition, some neurosyphilis patients in the U.S. who were treated with chloroquine suffered relapses attributed to the acquired resistance of the disease organisms (Jeffery, 1976).

In 1959 and 1960, resistance was documented in South America and Southeast Asia. Two employees of a geophysical company working on seismographic explorations in Colombia became very ill with falciparum malaria. One took sick in 1959, the other the following year. Both took chloroquine but neither responded. Both were flown to Dallas where they were hospitalized, and their progress was monitored closely. First, they were unsuccessfully treated with larger doses of chloroquine. Then other drugs were tried including primaquine, another recently developed synthetic, and quinine sulfate. Neither of those was effective. Eventually, the disease just ran its course, and both men survived (Moore and Lanier, 1961).

Before long, drug resistance was common in South Asia and Southeast Asia, particularly among remote forested hills along routes traveled by miners or traders. Many had dosed themselves with chloroquine, which was as common as aspirin. Mosquitoes and malaria were unavoidable. It would be easy to see how a disease organism might develop resistance to a drug that way. Then, as new replacement drugs appeared on the market, many of those quickly lost their power to cure malaria.

Did the resistance factor spread from region to region, as if it were a contagious disease? Some investigators thought "yes."

Or did resistance of the parasite to certain medicines actually emerge independently here and there? In other words, did falciparum malaria possess some inherent characteristics that allowed it to resist threatening substances? There appeared to be evidence for a "yes" there as well.

Scientists continued to find new evidence of inherent resistance. Two prominent scientists wrote: "... this type of refractoriness of malaria parasites to drugs does not reflect a recently acquired, recently detected, or unanticipated lack of responsiveness of the parasites to drugs, but, rather a long recognized inherent insensitivity on the part of certain forms of malaria parasites to certain agents"[8] (Powell and Tigertt, 1968).

Some scientists believed they had evidence that the resistance factor might not be portable. In an isolated, forested area in Madhya Pradesh, India, an outbreak of chloroquine-resistant falciparum malaria drew attention from health authorities. Yet, studies of the area did not reveal any excessive use or misuse of drugs. In fact, inhabitants had virtually no previous contact with outsiders, nor any access to health care providers (Sharma, et al., 1991).

Physicians in Nigeria believed they had witnessed another encounter with falciparum malaria that seemed to possess an inherent capacity for resistance to medicines. In that case, *falciparum* parasites were found to be resistant to the antimalarial drug mefloquine before the drug had been used in the region. The investigators interpreted the event as an example of malaria's inherent resistance to the medicine (Oduola, 1988). In other areas of the world, parasites had displayed what seemed

146

like instant drug resistance. In addition, as other new drugs were introduced, a new phrase was used for the problem. The evasive parasites were called "multi-resistant strains."[9] According to one scientist, by 1988, multiple drug-resistant strains of *P. falciparum* had been identified in virtually every country where that parasite was transmitted (Peters, 1992).

The development was bad news for health providers and drug manufacturers as well as victims of the disease. Incentives for creating new malaria medicines were dwindling, in spite of encouragement offered in 1961 in a WHO technical report on drugs for malaria. It said, "The clinician has at his disposal a complete series of effective drugs for the treatment of all stages of the disease..."

DDT Revisited

One profound setback followed another. Both the disease organism and its winged vector were defying the celebrated tools created to destroy them. About the time chloroquine-resistant malaria was appearing at widely separated locations, DDT-resistant mosquitoes were returning to areas that had been sprayed—areas that sponsors of the insecticide thought were safe.

By 1960, five years after WHO launched its massive, ambitious eradication campaign, the signs were undeniable. In many places, particularly in South Asia and Southeast Asia, mosquitoes had become more aggressive and widespread. More people were dying. Confidence in DDT was waning.

Not everyone was surprised. Farmers in California as early as 1906, for instance, had stopped using two insecticides against California scale insects when they realized that the crop pests had developed resistance to the substance (Perkins, 1982). Early DDT teams in the U.S. reported resistance to the chemical after several household applications. One WHO entomologist reported several cases of DDT-resistant mosquitoes from 1948 to 1955 in California, Florida, Tennessee and Hawaii in the U.S., and also in Greece, Java, Nigeria, Saudi Arabia, Korea, Trinidad, Egypt and Israel. The scientist predicted more widespread resistance in the future if the agency persisted with its spraying strategy (Busvine, 1956).

Some DDT field workers offered possible explanations for the setback. They suggested that local spray teams had diluted the product for their own profit. Or, perhaps the teams were neglecting to cover the entire assigned territory. Or they didn't understand their instructions. Or their reports were inaccurate.

But as the months and years passed, the gravity of the problem was becoming clear. In 1969, the World Health Assembly analyzed the deteriorating conditions and recommended that WHO change its course. Instead of its singular commitment to DDT for eradicating malaria everywhere, countries that had signed on for the DDT field projects were advised they could choose another strategy to address special needs, as long as they coordinated their decisions and actions with their project supervisors. Conditions continued to deteriorate.

What went wrong? A studied response that did not shirk responsibility came from Jose Najera, a physician specialized in public health and tropical medicine who worked for WHO between 1961 and 1992. His account of the eradication campaign and the missteps along the way appeared in the Bulletin of the World Health Organization in 1989. The title was "Malaria and the Work of WHO."

According to Najera, program planners calculated they could outrun the resistance factor. That is, they believed they could eradicate the mosquito faster than resistance could emerge (Najera, 1989). But planners were wrong.

In another gamble, planners decided they did not need to waste time with preliminary epidemiological surveys. But disregard of epidemiological data was like flying without compass. On that point also, planners reportedly calculated that the studies would be a waste since DDT was already spelling doom for the mosquitoes *(Ibid.)*. Or so they thought.

148

Some of the Scars

The failed DDT campaign left several scars. By rejecting the wisdom and experience of seasoned malariologists, WHO planners fostered the polarization of government health efforts into two branches of activity: science and fieldwork. Management and agency finances often obscured the mutual goals of all health workers, putting cross-cultural teamwork in jeopardy. One scientist reported that WHO policies had created a negative, anti-U.S. atmosphere among people from other countries who worked with Americans on other health initiatives.[10]

It was speculated however, that those negative attitudes might have been connected with the U.S. dominance of the entire malaria effort. Persons familiar with the activities of international health organizations have said that WHO's malaria policy was effectively determined and controlled by U.S.A.I.D. (United States Agency for International Development) and CDC.

The single-minded faith in DDT may have created another problem. Specialists knew that a large eradication campaign that left an endemic population unharmed was effectively doomed. One scientist said, "Throughout the world, support for further research into malaria, even that concerned with insecticides and chemotherapeutics, contracted swiftly. Worse still, the apparently imminent demise of a once important disease removed the necessity for training scientists in malariology" (Najera, 1989, quoting McGregor I.A., Malaria: Introduction, *British Medical Bulletin*, 1982, 38:2).

It was logical to suppose that the DDT campaign actually opened the door to an increased intensity of malaria. As mentioned earlier, adults in a stable endemic location could maintain immunity to malaria if they were reinfected every few years. It was like having periodic booster shots. That worked as long as the residents did not travel to another community where they were exposed to different strains and as long as visitors from other regions did not introduce new strains to the stable community.

When DDT temporarily eradicated a community's mosquitoes, many of the residents who missed their immunity "booster" would be susceptible to dangerous infections when the mosquitoes and the disease returned. After a few years, people who had been protected would be nonimmune and as vulnerable as young children. There was another potential problem. If the only mosquitoes that survived a series of sprayings had inherent resistance or possessed genes that could mutate into strong resistant populations quickly, WHO policy was in effect selectively breeding stronger and stronger malaria vectors.

Those trends, if valid, could account for the transmission pattern that evolved early in the DDT campaign. The mosquitoes seemed to get stronger and stronger, that is, more resistant to DDT. In those first several years DDT was remarkably effective in Ceylon, India and other places. Transmission of malaria dropped quickly and radically. But several years later the disease returned, more severe than ever. Actually, many distinguished malariologists from the U.S. and elsewhere never believed in the possibility of eradication under tropical conditions.

New Campaign Planned

By 1998, WHO was ready to launch a new massive antimalaria campaign, with the co-sponsorship of the World Bank, UNESCO and traditional donors. The strategy addressed old problems and new lessons connected with malaria control. Planners acknowledged that malaria was actually a local disease. Each endemic location was unique. Each epidemic was unique. Success depended on the ability of the health workers to understand the dynamics of the disease and create a specific strategy for each trouble spot. Decisions would be based on epidemiological evidence. Public health infrastructure and training would be improved. More money would be assigned to development of new drugs. After 43 years of disappointment, the unrealistic word "eradication" was discarded.

It might be difficult for future historians to understand why it took so long for international health authorities to give up on DDT. One historian had an explanation. Writing in 1978, Gordon Harrison said that it was not easy for WHO to abandon the goal that had been pursued so single-mindedly. He pointed out that WHO had tried for 14 years to eradicate malaria with DDT. He wrote: "WHO had pushed eradication with such zeal and held out for it such brilliant promise that its *amour propre*[11] argued desperately against retreat. So it gave way very slowly, with many a backward glance at what might have been and a particularly painful sense of failure" (Harrison, 1978).

---

[1] See table on page 125.

[2] A blood-dwelling animal parasite.

[3] *The Edwin Smith Papyrus* "probably the first scientific document in the history of medicine," was written by Impotep circa 3,000 BC and describes 48 surgical cases (Marti-Ibanez, 1961).

[4] The TVA projects inspired several successful drainage programs in Europe. They included the project conducted by American malariologist Lewis Hackett in Italy and the project managed by Italy's Mussolini in Pontine Marshes.

[5] An insect that prefers "lower animals" to humankind as a source of food.

[6] U.S. president Woodrow Wilson had proposed establishing the league at the end of the war. But the U.S. Congress rejected it. Consequently, the U.S. was not a member.

[7] See p. 96 for account of World War II.

[8] William Tigertt, director of the Walter Reed Army Institute of Research, at the time, and Robin Powell of the University of Chicago.

[9] Sometimes referred to as MRS.

[10] WHO was an international organization, affiliated with the United Nations. but the U.S. paid most of the operating funds.

[11] Self-esteem.

My first experiment was made upon a lad of the name of Phipps, in whose arm a little Vaccine Virus was inserted taken from the hand of a young woman who had been accidentally infected by a cow. Notwithstanding the resemblance which the pustule thus excited on the boy's arm bore to variolous inoculation, yet as the indisposition attending it was barely perceptible, I could scarcely persuade myself the patient was secure from the Smallpox. However, on his being inoculated some months afterwards, it proved that he was secure. This case inspired me with confidence, and as soon as I could again furnish myself with Virus from the Cow, I made an arrangement for a series of inoculations.

E. Jenner
The Origin of the Vaccine Inoculation, 1801
The event described took place on May 14, 1796
(Henderson, 1997)

Chapter 7
The Malaria Vaccine

EDWARD JENNER'S "variolous inoculation," later known as a vaccination, had been practiced in one way or an-other by ancient and modern cultures in many parts of the world. It was believed in some places that a small amount of a disease organism — maybe just part of a scab — might protect a person against the disease.

Since early times, the smallpox virus was a common killer just about everywhere. Large pustules disfigured the skin of survivors. Some people suspected a link between the sores on cows and the human disease. It certainly was a credible theory. Even during smallpox epidemics, milkmaids in the community kept their unblemished complexions. They seemed to be immune to the disease.

In Glasgow between 1783 and 1800, 50 percent of the children died before 10 years of age. Half of those deaths were due to smallpox. The disease then was the leading cause of blindness throughout Europe. But within three years after the new procedure was in use, vaccinations were being administered all across Europe, Asia and North America, and in 1979 the World Health Organization announced that smallpox had been eradicated from the whole world. No vaccine since Jenner's time was made available to the public so quickly or has been so effective.

The second human vaccination was developed to prevent another deadly viral disease, rabies. It was created by Louis Pasteur and was ready for use in 1855 (Henderson, 1997). Several other vaccines followed over the years, but no vaccine has ever been approved for use against a parasite, at least not by the end of the 20th century.

Why Not a Malaria Vaccine?

The odds had never been good for a malaria vaccine—that is, a reliable malaria vaccine like the smallpox vaccine that virtually all individuals everywhere could count on for long-term immunity. Malaria was not like smallpox, rabies, polio, measles, yellow fever and the rest. Each of those other diseases that were prevented with vaccines was caused by organisms with a consistent, predictable set of genes, hardly the way one could describe the malaria parasite.

Remember, the malaria parasite was a real animal, part of a classification of animals called *Protozoa*, or "first animals." They were really ancient. It was believed they took up residence in life forms that were humankind's earliest ancestors. The two, the parasite and the host, continued to evolve together, each adapting to the needs and threats of the other, and their evolution hadn't stopped. Their bonds seemed to be made to last.

Research Prospects

By about 1940, malaria was no longer a public health threat in the United States, which had become the primary funding source for medical research worldwide. Ten years later, labs in the U.S. and Europe were producing antimalaria drugs. But people soon became convinced that the sensational new insecticide DDT and the effective drug chloroquine erased the threat of malaria.

That dream didn't last long. By about 1960, the public was aware that malaria was returning. The parasite was developing resistance to the medicines, and mosquitoes were developing resistance to DDT. During that same period, microbiologists were becoming acquainted with a succession of new tools in their labs that were allowing them to investigate and manipulate minuscule cellular products. The prospects for a malaria vaccine seemed good.

HIGH TECHNOLOGY

- Improvements in the ***electron microscope*** allowed scientists to see things almost half a million times smaller than what was seen with the naked eye.
- New ***ultracentrifuges*** could spin 80,000 revolutions per minute, separating various minute components of substances under analysis.
- With ***X-ray crystallographic*** studies, scientists could define the structure of proteins and DNA by crystallizing them and bombarding them with electrons.
- The development of ***recombinant DNA techniques*** allowed manipulations of DNA and catapulted the malaria field into a new arena.
- A new technique called ***Polymerase Chain Reaction*** and its subsequent automation allowed scientists to examine the genetic material of a single cell in a relatively short time.

Scientists could then focus on the expanding frontiers of the inner functioning of the cells, DNA, genes, proteins and amino acids.

Every gene the parasite needed was in each cell. During the separate stages in the life cycle, however, it utilized only certain unique genes — that is, unique to the needs of that stage. By selecting new genes and abandoning old ones, the malaria parasite was able to perform a large variety of activities. The genes that were no longer needed could be turned off. New genes with new instructions were turned on, among them genes for the appropriate antigens.

In their new labs and with new support from optimistic sponsors, microbiologists could dissect the malaria parasite and look at its parts. They could examine the amino acids within the proteins and probe right into the cell's nucleus where they could see the strands of DNA, the "blueprint" that contained all the instructions for the cell.

The DNA with its sequences of genes was spread out in the form of two twisted strands like the rails of a ladder with rungs linking them. That was the "double helix" identified by scientists in the 1950s. The familiar drawing in the scientists' model looked like a neat structure built from children's construction toys. In images captured by the electron microscope, DNA looked like a messy ball of thin ribbon the cat was playing with.

Only four nucleic acids formed the bases of the seemingly simple structure, but in their combinations those molecules provided an apparently endless diversity of information. The DNA from the nucleus of a single human cell, for instance, could hold information equivalent to a library of thousands of books. Scientists were surprised to learn just how accessible the strands of DNA were, and how easily they could be cut and spliced with enzymes to open a new treasure of opportunities for genetic engineering. Opportunities included designing a new malaria vaccine.

Considering how much scientists learned and accomplished, it seemed incredible that any disease organism was safe. But mysteries prevailed, those mysteries about the parasite and the immune system, and about the particularly arcane evolutionary pathways that linked the two.

New Strategies

Another boost to vaccine research in the technology-charged 1960s was the new talent entering the field. One pioneer of vaccine research was Dr. Ruth Nussenzweig at New York University School of Medicine, whose early work was in collaboration with her husband, Dr. Victor Nussenzweig. They came to New York from Sao Paulo, Brazil, in the 1960s, when it was already assumed that any malaria vaccine would have to target just one of the parasite's stages, or one stage at a time.

The Nussenzweigs concentrated on the sporozoite stage of falciparum malaria, in some ways then and later a logical choice. That stage was the first link between the malaria parasite and its human host. The infected host wasn't even sick yet, so a successful sporozoite vaccine would prevent the disease.

Another reason for targeting sporozoites was that there weren't many of them, compared with the multimillions of parasites in the merozoite stage that followed. In addition, the sporozoite looked like a simple creature. Its surface proteins were large, covering the cell in folds, and all the sporozoites had the same antigenic composition. Those advantages seemed to outweigh the one apparent disadvantage, which was the fact that a sporozoite vaccine would have to work fast with 100 percent accuracy. The sporozoite was only exposed to antibodies of the human immune system for a period of minutes; it took the sporozoite less than an hour from the time it was injected with mosquito's saliva into the victim's capillaries until the time it squirmed into the relative safety of the liver. If just one sporozoite escaped, that one could multiply into enough merozoites to cause a full-blown, possibly fatal, attack of malaria.

The Nussenzweig team had to work with sporozoites harvested by hand. They dissected infected mosquitoes, took live sporozoites from their mouthparts and irradiated them so they could not reproduce. The irradiated parasites still had their surface proteins intact to perform their designated tasks, like displaying antigens. A vaccine was in the making.

In 1967, the experimental vaccine was ready. It was administered to laboratory mice, which gained protection from infection. In 1973 and 1974, other research teams in collaboration with the Nussenzweigs used irradiated sporozoite vaccines on human volunteers, who were protected when they later were exposed to malaria. Further trials had to wait until a process could be found to produce sporozoites artificially. It was impossible to collect enough of the parasites by dissecting mosquitoes one at a time.

Subunit Vaccine Raises Hopes

The Nussenzweigs soon learned more about the single protein that covered each cell of the sporozoite. The protein consisted of a chain of several hundred amino acids arranged in patterns. The Nussenzweigs called it the CS protein, and it quickly became one of the most widely studied proteins in laboratories throughout the world. Next, Ruth Nussenzweig cloned human antibodies to the CS protein, opening a new direction in vaccine research. From then on, a steady supply of the cloned antibodies was available for research.

C. Nigel Godson of the New York University Medical Center discovered ways to identify the specific sequence of amino acids on the CS protein that the cloned antibodies could most easily recognize. The sequence or subunit had a simple pattern, repeated frequently. The scientists assumed that the sequence was important in the functioning of the protein. They determined also that the subunit was indeed setting off alarms in the human immune system. That is, antibodies were alerted.

That amino acid sequence was selected for a new subunit vaccine, the first of its kind. Early trials brought good results, apparently confirming that certain very small pieces of a disease organism could indeed stimulate antibodies. The subunit was mass-produced and freedom from malaria seemed within reach.

But as the trials progressed, it became clear that the antibodies summoned by those subunit vaccines were not providing reliable protection against the disease; sometimes they worked, and sometimes they did not. Several new techniques and materials were tried, but the results were basically the same. The presence of antibodies did not guarantee protection against the disease. A pattern was appearing that would thwart researchers for many years.

Several reasons were offered for the disappointing outcome. It seemed as if the parasite tricked the immune system. But how? Were the parasites creating decoys so the antibodies missed the target? Were the antibodies lost in the upper folds of the proteins? Was that particular subunit actually the best target, or was there another more obscure subunit that was really more important? Or were the antibodies summoned by the subunit just too slow to establish immunity in the narrow window of opportunity before the sporozoites moved into the liver?

Another question that could not be avoided concerned the fact that even natural antibodies to malaria stimulated by hordes of whole live parasites delivered in the spittle of the mosquito did not provide total immunity. Was it really logical to assume that antibodies stimulated artificially by a fragment of the parasite would be more successful? Many scientists said "yes," it would be logical that a subunit vaccine could do the job if researchers found the perfect delivery system, used enough valid components, and combined them in just the right way. Other scientists were not so sure.

Scientist Jumps the Gun

One researcher at the U.S. Naval Medical Research Institute in Bethesda, Maryland, learned just how unreliable and potentially dangerous vaccine trials can be. In 1987, Dr. Stephen Hoffman, head of the Institute's malaria program, and his colleagues were particularly hopeful about a candidate vaccine for sporozoites that they were developing. So the team decided to test it on themselves. Hoffman recalled, "We were quite enthusiastic at the time and in retrospect perhaps a little bit naive" (Hoffman, 1988).

The volunteers knew in advance that the live parasites that would infect them were sensitive to chloroquine. Anyone who got sick could be safely treated. Each volunteer was inoculated with the experimental vaccine. Then they established through examination of their own blood that the vaccine did indeed induce an antibody response. They were ready to "challenge" themselves with live parasites. The challenge was delivered by *Anopheles* mosquitoes infected by *P. falciparum* sporozoites and hungry for blood. They were carried in a small container like an ice cream carton with a piece of gauze over the top.

Each volunteer placed the carton upside down over his arm and let the mosquitoes bite. If some of the insects didn't oblige, the volunteers replaced them and kept the process going until each man had been infected by at least five mosquitoes.

They then waited to see if at last they had found the right formula for successful protection. Several of the men developed symptoms of malaria, and their blood tested positive for the disease. The trial vaccine had not protected them. Those men were treated with chloroquine, and they recovered.

Hoffman and two others, however, tested negative for malaria. They had had enough antibodies to lead them to think that they were protected. Ten days after the challenge with captive mosquitoes, Hoffman had to fly to California to give a speech about malaria. On the eleventh day the classic symptoms began. He thought at first he just had the flu. A doctor tested Hoffman's blood for malaria parasites, but found none.

Since he was part of a monitored vaccine trial, Hoffman was determined to delay treatment until a diagnosis was confirmed.

160

The next day he was critically ill, with a temperature of 104 degrees Fahrenheit, violent chills and vomiting. He felt as if he were going to die. But still no parasites were discernible on his blood slide, and Hoffman still refused treatment. Finally his doctor was able to get a positive blood smear, and he started Hoffman on chloroquine — just in time. He was becoming jaundiced. The next day his skin turned yellow with jaundice, but he recovered without complications.

The episode didn't spoil Hoffman's enthusiasm for his vaccine quest. Nor did the realization that the antibodies stimulated thus far by the vaccines weren't blocking infection. Some obviously were slipping into the liver, off-limits for human antibodies.

On to the Liver

Some vaccine researchers shifted their attention to the last period of sporozoites when they were in the liver. Stopping the malaria parasites while they were in the liver was an exciting prospect. Then the parasite could not cause disease and could not reproduce. But the job would have to be absolutely perfect, considering how fast those sporozoites multiplied. Just one escaped parasite could soon create enough progeny to kill the host (Hedstrom, 1997).

Some scientists chose to try to enlist help from one of the other kind of immune agents that might be mobilized to function inside the liver. Those were the "killer cells" of the cellular immune system, which attacked and engulfed just about any foreign substance they could reach.

In 1991, Hoffman and his colleagues believed they had found a way to fortify the CS vaccine with a protein to stimulate the killer cells to attack sporozoites in the liver. The process reportedly worked in laboratory mice, a success story that made new celebratory headlines for malaria research. Then researchers around the world began looking for an adaptation of the mouse victory that would be successful in human beings (Hoffman, 1991).

In a way, that technique might be called a long shot. The killer cells didn't act very fast, and sporozoites didn't stay in the liver long, only for 10–12 days. By the time the killer cells recognized the enemy and began their attack, the enemy could be gone. Then the sporozoites would be free to enter the blood, wearing their new identities as merozoites (Taubes, 1997).

Focus on Merozoites

Work to create a vaccine against the merozoite stage of the *falciparum* parasite began in 1976 with a pivotal discovery by Dr. William Trager at Rockefeller University in New York City. He developed a technique for growing merozoites in a culture of human blood, giving researchers their first easy access to that stage for vaccine experiments.

Merozoites that emerged from the liver were teardrop shaped, much larger than sporozoites and much more complex. Their duties were crucial. Each merozoite was in charge of orchestrating about 3,000 antigens, most of which did not alert antibodies. Merozoites had to create the gametocytes that would perpetuate their species, and they had to defend themselves from human immune agents. Their programmed mass invasions of red blood cells gave them energy to fulfill their obligations. But it also made their hosts very sick and sometimes killed them.

Scientists developing vaccine strategies were confronting a tangle of problems in identifying the antigens, or proteins, and their assigned functions. Self-defense was one of the merozoites' responsibilities. One way to protect themselves was to disguise their critical surface proteins, the proteins that had responsibilities for critical functions. The cell could disguise proteins by creating a smoke screen effect with the otherwise worthless proteins. Sometimes the surface proteins would mimic antibodies to sidetrack an imminent attack from human immune agents. Or they could display an excessively large quantity of pseudo-antigens to trick the immune system into expending an excessive response. An excessive volume of unneeded human immune agents might threaten the life of the host.

Scientists began looking for surface proteins that might have a specific role in triggering an immune reaction from the host. They were also looking for more details about the novel mechanisms created by the parasite to prevent the human immune response from achieving total success in the battle.

By the end of the 20th century, scientists still had not learned how to recognize which antigens were relevant to the organism's survival. There were other important details, however, that were being discovered.

One observation attracted the attention of researchers. It occurred when a fresh merozoite prepared to attack a red blood cell, as observed under an electron microscope.

The parasites that bumped into red cells seemed to reorient themselves in a unique way. Once the parasite had reoriented and formed a junction with the red cell, it extruded certain contents from its apical end or the tip of the teardrop that were believed to influence the red cell. The cell under attack seemed to cave in, assuming a submissive posture to facilitate the enemy's invasion. The blood cell then created a kind of pocket by which the parasite could slip right in; finally it closed the opening, allowing the parasite to devour hemoglobin (Hall, 1992). It was speculated that the unusual bond between the two represented the evolution of the cell when the earth was very young (Hyde, 1990).

Even if a perfect vaccine were developed — like the yellow fever vaccine — microbiologists probably would continue to explore the relationship of the malaria parasite and its host's immune resources, just for the sake of pure science.

Targeting Gametocytes

After a couple of weeks, some of the merozoites interrupted their preoccupation with devouring hemoglobin from the host's red blood cells and assumed the third and final stage of the parasite's life cycle. They became male and female gametocytes. As the reader knew, that was the sexual stage, also known as the transmission stage. When a mosquito bit an infected victim, gametocytes then rode along with the rest of the blood meal into the mosquito's stomach. That's where fertilization took place, resulting in thousands of sporozoites that would travel up to the mosquito's saliva to await their trip to a new host.

A successful gametocyte vaccine would not benefit the human host, but it might prevent infection among other people in the community. Some people called the concept an "altruistic" vaccine. It was speculated that a gametocyte vaccine might be used in combination with vaccines against other stages, in a kind of multicomponent or "cocktail" vaccine.

The idea of packaging two or more vaccines together was appealing to some researchers. If the vaccine missed catching the sporozoites, for instance, it would have another chance in the liver or in the blood stream, or maybe inside the victim of the sporozoite's offspring. By the mid-1990s, several research teams were assembling such packages. Scientists at the labs of the Walter Reed Army Institute of Research (WRAIR) in Washington, D.C., were experimenting with vaccine packages loaded with seven separate malaria genes (Ballou, 1994).

Over at the Naval Medical Research Institute, not far from the WRAIR labs, a team of molecular biologists was trying to create a new malaria vaccine based on a very new approach. It was a DNA vaccine, using a tiny strip of DNA, the twisted threads of nucleic acids that carried coded information relating to the responsibilities of each cell. Scientists had learned that the strips of DNA were more durable than they appeared. They could be cut easily, used for different purposes and stored for future use.

The possibility that DNA could be used as a vaccine to protect people from disease was realized in 1990. Three years later it was used as a flu vaccine. Then researchers at several establishments were experimenting with DNA vaccines against colon cancer, hepatitis B, AIDS, cutaneous T-cell lymphoma and herpes. Several investigators believed the new techniques might lead to a successful malaria vaccine.

Each new "breakthrough" in the laboratory shed new light on parasitic relationships in general and on the very specific events that took place in the different phases of the antagonism between the malaria parasite and its human host. No one could guess when or if any of the new work would benefit the millions of sufferers, and researchers feared funders were getting impatient.

New Vaccine is Tested in the Field

Meanwhile, during the period when molecular biologists from industrialized countries faced a series of stalemates and other disappointments, a biologist in Colombia was creating his own vaccine. It was the first malaria vaccine to graduate from the laboratory to field trials on human subjects, the first synthetic vaccine, and the first created by a scientist from the developing world. The creator was Manuel Patarroyo, and he called his vaccine SPf66. Patarroyo and SPf66 were names that would arouse unparalleled controversy for several years (Riley, 1995).

Some people pointed out that it was not completely understood what made the Patarroyo vaccine work. U.S. malariologist Ripley Ballou said the vaccine was "not understood at all." But he said, "For probably 95 percent of the vaccines we have gotten — licensed vaccines in the United States — no one can tell you exactly how they work." He said most of the earlier vaccines were developed empirically. "We found something that worked and then we could make it reproducibly and then showed that it worked." That was the way Patarroyo worked.

In contrast, 99 percent of modern vaccines against malaria were done with "designer methodology." Ballou explained, "We have an idea why it should work because we know what antigen is involved. We know the region of the antigen that is involved. We have a proposed mechanism of action. And then we try to construct a vaccine based around that" (Ballou, 1994).

Patarroyo's Strategy

Patarroyo started with parasites from human beings who were infected with malaria but who weren't sick.

His new vaccine consisted of synthetic peptides, or small bits of proteins, from two stages of the parasite — the sporozoite and the merozoite. Health professionals had known for a long time that many people in an endemic community had substances in their blood giving them temporary or partial immunity to malaria. Could such substances be applied to other people for protection? Patarroyo was betting that they could. His strategy was not much different from Jenner's search for a smallpox vaccine starting with milkmaids who had acquired immunity from cowpox.

Patarroyo's production process was tedious. He used antibodies from immune persons to identify proteins in the malaria parasite that looked as if they were active in the immune process. He collected 22 proteins in all and then injected them into monkeys collected from the rain forests. From the monkeys' blood he identified four proteins that looked promising. He sequenced those four and from them reconstructed dozens of short fragments, or peptides. The next step was with monkeys again, more than 1,000 of them. Patarroyo used them to test his synthetic peptides individually or in combinations until he was able to choose three for a trial vaccine.

The Trials

Were the tests successful? That was debatable, and the debate got hot. Part of the story was told in the trial results.[1] In 1985–86 in Bogota, Colombia, trials in monkeys demonstrated that the vaccine was safe, that it stimulated immunity, and that it was partially protective against the disease. The following year the vaccine was partially effective in trials with nine soldiers. That was when Patarroyo publicly announced his achievement.

Within the following six years at least 12 field trials on the product were held in Colombia, Brazil, Equador and Venezuela on a variety of subjects, including monkeys and human beings. The results were mixed, reaching as high as 55 percent, 67 percent and 82 percent subjects protected.

Later trials in Africa and in Thailand were not so encouraging. In Gambia in 1994, 600 children 6–11 months old were vaccinated. No protection was noted. The next year in Idete, Tanzania, 586 children 1–5 years old were vaccinated, and 31 percent protection was recorded. The following year in Kilombero, Thailand, 1,250 children 2–16 years old were vaccinated. No protection was noted (Maurice, 1995).

Significance

Sifting the results for substantive information was a challenge. The scores of two large field trials at widely separated regions were similar, 31 percent efficacy in Tanzania and 37 percent in Colombia. Most observers used the former number when characterizing the potential of the product. But specialists pointed out that comparisons of the various results had no value.

The geographic settings were widely different. Latin America in general had only seasonal transmission of the disease. The locations in Africa and Thailand had year- around endemic or hyperendemic malaria. There was no consistency in the ages of the volunteers nor in the sizes of the groups tested. They did not share common protocols for monitoring outcomes. There was no indication that mistakes were made at any one of the locations. But the figures did not furnish any information that would help in forming new strategies.

Results from the trials in Thailand had been awaited with high expectations, then regarded with grave disappointment. That location was just inside the border with Myanmar (formerly Burma) in a highly endemic area with a history of heavy presence of drug-resistant strains of the disease. A total of 1,200 children 2–16 years old took part. No protection against malaria was noted. The site of the study was a refugee camp known as Shoklo, maintained by the Thai government. The occupants were ethnic Karen Burmese who had been displaced from Myanmar by the government there. The residents were not permitted to have visas. They could neither travel freely in Thailand nor go back to their home country. For the purposes of conducting vaccine trials, it was a most reliable location. Women among the refugee community were trained to assist in administering the test.

Reactions Varied Widely

The bulk of results for the 10 years of trials drew dramatically divided responses from the public. Officials, health professionals and citizenry from Colombia, elsewhere in Latin America, and from a few other locations were exuberant. A visitor to Patarroyo's office said the scientist's shelves were "sagging with prizes," at least 53 of them (Maurice, 1995).

As early as 1994, Patarroyo was receiving urgent requests for his vaccine from other countries. Bolivia asked for 600 doses and Zaire (now the Democratic Republic of Congo) wanted 10 million. Indonesia sought permission to produce the vaccine in its own production plant. An offer to buy $300 million worth of the vaccine came from an oil-drilling firm in Kenya. Five countries with endemic malaria reportedly joined in a plan to vaccinate a million people in massive field trials in a project to be supported by a $3.8 million grant from the government of Spain (*Ibid.*).

Patarroyo was greeted with cheers when he appeared at an international conference in Brazil. Ruth Nussenzweig, the other Latin American hero of vaccine research, was there as well, quietly nodding and deferring to the new star (Author's observation, 1990).

Observers from industrial countries were not uniformly supportive about Patarroyo's results. The rounded out efficacy figure of 31 percent was not really a good score for a vaccine. Some people believed that the score for the trials in Tanzania was actually too high, considering that only a small number of malaria episodes were reported.

The prestigious medical journal *Lancet* editorialized that the trials were a failure and that further trials using the same materials were not warranted. Paul-Henri Lambert, chief of WHO's vaccine research and development unit, said "A 31 percent rate is in a gray zone, at the limit of ineffectiveness." Roy Widdus, a vaccine expert with the U.S. Public Health Service, said that a 31 percent level of protection "will not reduce transmission of the disease to a significant extent." He said, that would be similar to what one might expect from a medicine that provided only partial success, with the disease continuing to survive as a public health problem.

Others defended a 31 percent efficacy and supported wide use of the product. Spanish epidemiologist Pedro Alonso, who was a member of the trial team in Tanzania, urged approval of the vaccine. He said, "Try telling the villagers in Africa that they're going to have to wait while they watch their children die from malaria." As quoted in *Science*, he said, "A 31 percent efficacy is not a lot, but you have to relate this figure to the severity of the disease. For a disease that causes 300 million clinical episodes a year, (the vaccine) will prevent at least 100 million episodes" (Maurice, 1995).

Some prominent U.S. malaria specialists supported the Patarroyo vaccine and supported, as well, a commitment to continue vaccine research. Robert Gwadz, of the U.S. National Institutes of Health, said, "We're not talking about polio-type vaccines, where you get immunized and you never get the disease… We're probably talking about vaccines that eliminate mortality and significantly reduce the level of sickness association with the disease."

William E. Collins and Altaf A. Lal of the U.S. Centers for Disease Control and Prevention appealed for sustained funding for vaccine research, in spite of the SPf66 results. They also urged that more consistency should be applied to the fulfillment of criteria for the graduation of vaccine candidates from animal to human trials. Then more potential problems could be identified before the human trials began. The two also urged researchers and sponsors not to give up the concepts of SPf66. They said, "The field failure of the SPf66 vaccine does not mean that malaria vaccines are a failed concept." They also said that untold millions of children in generations to come could die from malaria if vaccine studies were stopped (Collins, 1996).

The comments were reminiscent of language used on countless occasions since the scientific community took responsibility for eradicating the disease back in the late 1940s. The assumption was that the only way to deal with the disease was with "breakthroughs" in science. That attitude, however, was beginning to lose its currency, and some scientists had already lost faith in vaccines.

A biologist from Scotland, Eleanor Riley, summed up the unwieldy assortment of figures and comments (Riley, 1995). She said the concerns could be divided into two categories, scientific arguments and political arguments. In the former category, the debate centered on whether the vaccine really worked and, if so, how. In that debate the lines were sharply drawn, with no consensus in sight. Sometime in the future, however, a retrospective view of vaccine development in the last part of the 20th century might settle on the real significance of Patarroyo's achievements. For the political arguments, Riley listed several topics. They included funding and assessment of the program, the speed at which the vaccine progressed to large field trials, and "ethical issues regarding widescale use of a vaccine with limited efficacy."

For assessments, Riley agreed with others who recommended that any future trials of malaria vaccines should be broader in scope. They should include many more participants from several regions, with uniform guidelines and central management for planning, implementation and monitoring. Riley also said, "In the future we should exercise caution when publicizing vaccine studies and should avoid the temptation of promising a vaccine within a given period of time."

The topic of "ethical issues" was laden with grave implications, especially for people in Africa. Scientists said that wide use of a malaria vaccine of limited efficacy "could accelerate the emergence of new forms not susceptible to host immunity" (Hyde, 1990). What a sad burden to inflict on a population already threatened by polio, measles, tuberculosis, tetanus and yellow fever — diseases that had been cured or controlled in most of the world. The same population was threatened as well by rampant AIDS.

---

[1] Standard procedures for field testing of vaccines in human subjects required three stages: a safety test; a test to determine if the material was immunogenic, that is, did the vaccine stimulate an immune response from the volunteer; and finally, did that response actually protect the volunteer from the disease?

171

"What a paradox! Man with his incredible machines and his streamlined science, stricken each year in millions because he fails to outwit a mosquito carrying death in its spittle!"

Paul Russell[1], 1943 (Russell, 1943).

Chapter 8
New Paths, Old Paths

A
LMOST FIFTY YEARS after Russell's exclamation, malaria death rates were rising, and hopes for a scientific breakthrough that would save the world from malaria were fading but not abandoned. Microbiologists and public health specialists pursued new paths, conceding that their original goal was far more challenging than they had anticipated. The last part of the 20th century could be characterized as an interlude of humility and reflection for malaria science.

Perhaps the interlude may be used for a review of the status of several initiatives:

- As new techniques became available, microbiologists pursued leads pointing to possible illumination of those links between the human immune system and the wily parasite.
- Epidemiological surveys were uncovering patterns of disease or patterns of resistant strains not previously recognized.
- New antimalarials based on ancient medicine were being examined in a modern context.

- Recommendations were mounting for strategies linking the wisdom of communities with the most malaria experience to the wisdom of scientists applying the new theories and techniques.
- Some scientists and other interested persons were exploring the ethical issues that arose when scientists from industrial countries created and tested their products in a third world setting.

The issue of ethics might be a good place to start. Many specialists still wanted to address issues left over from the disappointing trials of the Patorroyo vaccine. They included the conflict between scientists from rich countries and poor people of the developing countries.

The issues were debated at a symposium on ethics and public health in 1992 sponsored by the Institute of Medicine and the American Society of Tropical Medicine and Hygiene.[2] The speakers were Michele Barry of Yale University in the U.S. and Malcolm Molyneux of the Liverpool School of Tropical Medicine in the U.K. Several of the questions were based on the Nuremberg Code and the Helsinki Declaration.[3]

Exceptions for Malaria?

BARRY asked if there was a justification for relaxing those ethical principles when conducting trials of malaria vaccines.

MOLYNEAUX: "Malaria is mainly a disease of developing countries. Most of the million or more people who die of malaria every year are young children in endemic areas. It is therefore in these areas that most clinical trials of drugs, and in due course vaccines, must be carried out. Local health services cannot be expected to have the money, time or personnel to mount studies of drugs or vaccines without the collaboration of scientists from industrial nations. Malaria is therefore a disease that requires for its study a bridging between cultures, a sharing of very different kinds of expertise between nations."

Informed Consent

BARRY: "Yet a number of ethical difficulties must arise in connection with clinical trials in developing nations. The first has to do with the willingness of subjects to take part in trials. The Nuremberg Code requires that individuals should only be subjected to biomedical research if they, or their responsible representative, give consent freely and without coercion, having been adequately informed of the nature and purpose of the study. Taking the latter point first, Dr. Molyneux, can an African villager involved in one of your studies fully understand your reasons for wanting to enroll her unconscious child in a study in which he may or may not be given an additional antimalarial drug? Is she able to make a free assessment of the possible risks versus possible benefits, before giving her consent in that setting?"

MOLYNEAUX: " 'Informed consent' is a problem anywhere. In a consensus conference in this country, 79 of 92 participants considered that the obtaining of informed consent was problematic because patients or surrogates could not fully understand the implications of a formal clinical trial. When we work in a foreign culture, we make sure that potential participants, or their surrogates, receive as clear an explanation as possible in their own language, given to them by a member of the trial team who belongs to that culture. The explanation must be made with due understanding of the individual's educational background, and in the light of local concepts of health and disease. Individuals may not understand the science of the study, but it is quite possible for the choice to be presented in a way that they can understand. As Ajayi, has said it is false to equate illiteracy with the inability to take decisions."[4]

Who's to Blame?

BARRY: "Isn't it true in some cultures people have ideas about health and disease that are incompatible with a scientific explanation? For example, the belief that disease is caused by an aggrieved enemy or ancestor, or that to remove a blood-sample is to rob a person of essential vitality?"

MOLYNEAUX: "People's beliefs about the causes of disease sometimes reduce recruitment to trials or may make them impossible. But in drug trials, the very fact that a patient has come for treatment indicates a willingness to try a scientific remedy. Many people are suspicious of our attempts to explain disease. (In the case of malaria their suspicions are well founded: although we know about the parasite, we ourselves have very little understanding of the pathogenic mechanisms of the *disease*.) Nevertheless, investigators must remain sensitive to differences in the way they and their patients understand disease; discussion and explanation may be necessary at intervals during a study, not only at the beginning."

Consent and Enrollment

BARRY: "Whatever the setting, in both industrial and developing communities, participants in a trial ultimately place their trust in the investigator and believe that he or she is acting in their best interest. Yet there clearly have to be safeguards to ensure that enrollment into a study is culturally comprehensible and not coercive. What about the act of consent itself? Consent as we understand it requires the decision of a free, autonomous individual — a person able to decide for herself without constraint or undue pressure from others. Is it not true that in many cultures, individual autonomy may be a dynamic system involving the family, group or village? How meaningful is the individual's "informed consent" in such circumstances?"

MOLYNEAUX: "For many trials, especially those which will take place within the village setting (for example, vaccine trials), decisions about participation are likely to be made at the level of the extended family, village or even tribal authority. In smallpox vaccine trials and trials of insecticide-spraying investigators reported that once the tribal leaders or elders, or the village as a whole, agreed to a study, it was rare for any individual to decline."

Imperialism

BARRY: "So, community involvement may be as important as individual consent in some cultural settings, yet obviously should not override or substitute for an individual's refusal to participate. Given the enormous gap in the level of scientific knowledge between the investigators and the people to be studied, is there not great potential for a kind of paternalistic scientific imperialism in malaria trials? What safeguards are there to ensure that scientists are not able to manipulate subjects into participation in studies that might not be in the subjects' best interests?"

MOLYNEAUX: "Almost every country now has its own scientific and ethical review board, to which every proposed trial must be submitted. In these committees, professionals or laypersons within the country may question the justification for a study or the benefit that the results are likely to bring to their own people. There may also be local ethical committees in the hospital or district in which a study is to be done. The existence of these local controls on scientific activity ensures that the proposal has been sanctioned by representatives of the people to be studied. The consenting individual is then placing her trust as much in her own countrymen as in the outsider."

Expectations

BARRY: "Yet often local review or ministry review boards can be responding to political pressures, foreign exchange or the interests of an elite. Double safeguards of both host and recipient independent review may mitigate this problem. What about the subtle pressure on individuals or groups to take part in studies; pressures that might flout the Helsinki requirement for freedom from coercion? I'm thinking, for example, of the extra clinical care that a mother might expect her child to receive if the child is admitted to a malaria-treatment study that provides not only a trial drug but also intensive care by the research team."

MOLYNEAUX: "In many cultures patients see their relationship with a healer in terms of a contract, and it is entirely reasonable that the contract should be mutually beneficial. The fact that there will be benefits in the form of health care for those entering a particular study is an appropriate part of the contract. It would be unreasonable to expect people to take part in a controlled trial, to put up with the additional sampling or interviewing involved, to have a 50 percent chance of receiving a placebo with no potential benefit whatsoever, and yet to have no additional compensation for taking part. In a field study, such as a vaccine trial, requiring the regular clinical evaluation of those who participate, clinical investigators cannot ignore other medical problems that their patients develop, and some general service may have to be offered. In practice it is usually logistically impossible to offer such services to the entire community; they may have to be offered as part of the contract to those who enroll in the study."

Harmful Effects?

BARRY: "Yet it is important to recognize that such services may reflect subtle pressure on an individual to enroll in a study. Leaving the difficult subject of informed consent, I'd like to consider the Hippocratic dictum — *primum non nocere*[5] — in relation to clinical trials in malaria. The Helsinki Declaration emphasizes that during the investigation of human subjects, the interest of science and society should never take precedence over consideration of the individual's well-being. If we consider trials of a malaria vaccine, is it possible that while a campaign may reduce transmission and benefit the community as a whole, the vaccinated individual may, as artificial immunity wanes, become more susceptible to severe malaria thereafter than he was before being vaccinated?"

MOLYNEAUX: "In any vaccine trial this possibility will have to be considered carefully. In the preliminary studies it should be possible to follow recipients closely, to detect any increased susceptibility with time and to provide effective treatment for malarial illness. The larger question is whether a successful vaccination programme would convert an area which has holoendemic[6], stable malaria into one which is subject to epidemic, unstable malaria, where many persons, both vaccinated and unvaccinated, may become susceptible to severe disease."

Precautions Applied

BARRY: "Thus, ongoing monitoring of malaria transmission in vaccinated areas will be crucial and will need to be supported after preliminary studies.

With all drug trials in developing nations, there is a danger that drugs which have not yet passed the stringent safety requirements of industrial nations might be used in populations with less developed regulatory mechanisms."

MOLYNEAUX: "This has happened quite often, in general therapeutic practice as well as in research. But it doesn't *need* to happen. Investigators should have to satisfy not only the scrutiny of host-country scientific and ethical committees, but also the requirements of both the collaborating institution and the donor of financial support."

Safety and Pregnancy

BARRY: "Yet, for example, malaria has high morbidity and mortality in pregnant women, a group that is virtually impossible to test in the United States for any new drug. Some of the earlier mefloquine studies which demonstrated the drug's safety during pregnancy were done by a U.S. agency in a developing nation, yet the drug was subsequently not released in the U.S. for use during pregnancy because of potential teratogenicity.[7] Should U.S. investigators be performing drug or vaccine studies on a population that would not be allowed to be tested here in the U.S.?"

MOLYNEAUX: "You said that malaria during pregnancy has a high morbidity; efficacious and safe drugs are desperately needed. We should remember that U.S. investigators must submit their research protocols for independent ethical review within their home country as well as in the host country, and the ethical standards applied are equally stringent wherever the work is to be done. The early mefloquine studies were subject to this process. The Food and Drug Administration (FDA) in the United States will, however, rarely license a drug for use in pregnancy without extensive human data. These data for malaria can only be collected in developing nations and sufficient data have not yet been gathered. The requirements of the FDA for licensing a drug in the U.S. are not the same as those that justify trials, and as long as ethical committees approve, trials should continue. The clinical problems are great, and we will not solve them by doing nothing."

Justice in Distribution

BARRY: "Clinical problems may be great, yet we must exercise consistent ethical standards in addressing them. I'd like to move on now to the principle of justice, which is that neither the benefits nor the burdens of research should be unjustly distributed. In other words, if the burden of preliminary trials of a drug or vaccine is to be borne by communities in malarious areas, the benefits of the resulting knowledge should be available to the same communities. Studies in a developing country may prove that a product is highly effective, but the knowledge may be useless to that country, if it cannot afford to buy supplies of the product. Meanwhile the richer world may have gained useful information for its travellers or soldiers. Would this not be a violation of the principle of justice?"

MOLYNEAUX: "Studies should be designed so that the host country can benefit from what is learned. But sometimes the benefit may not be immediate. For example, a successful trial may lead to a product becoming steadily cheaper as it is produced on a large scale, as happened with chloroquine. Some trials actually prove the *lack* of efficacy of a commonly used treatment, as in the studies that showed dexamethasone to be of no value in the treatment of cerebral malaria."

Sustaining Benefits

BARRY: "Yet in order to be ethically responsible, collaborative trials in developing nations should address the health priorities of the host country and not divert resources or manpower from more pressing health needs in order to study a question perhaps of more interest to the Western collaborator. It seems particularly possible that a malaria vaccine, although tested in the field in populations in endemic areas, might then be of greater benefit to the investigators than to the investigated. It may be easy to give a vaccine to travellers from rich nations but economically and logistically difficult to administer it to entire populations in poorer countries."

MOLYNEAUX: "This is a strong possibility. What is more likely is that a new vaccine will be introduced with enthusiasm but it will not be possible to sustain its distribution over time in areas in need of it. If a successful vaccine is developed, developed nations will need to devote considerable assistance, in funds and facilities, to help developing countries to sustain vaccination programmes. It will be unethical if rich nations fail to do this."

"Smash and Grab"

BARRY: "There is another aspect of justice which we should consider. It concerns not the population at risk of malaria, but the scientists and professional providers of health in countries where malaria is a major endemic disease. They too are at risk of exploitation. Is there any guarantee that when research studies are done by outside teams, some expertise is passed on to members of the host nation who have to remain and continue to work in their own country?"

MOLYNEAUX: "The World Health Organization's Training in Disease Research (TDR) programme aims to strengthen the capability of host countries to do research. Funds are given to promote collaborative work which includes a training component. All research — and indeed all service programmes in which rich and poor collaborate — should include a strong training function, so that the host country inherits not only the results of research but the capacity to identify and effectively study its own problems. It is all too common for an outside team to practice 'smash and grab' research, gathering data of interest to themselves or of benefit to their careers, and then disappearing without allowing their hosts the opportunity to participate in or carry forward the work, much less to benefit from it."

Compelling Needs

BARRY: "Clearly there are complexities, both ethical and logistic, in studying malaria. Our expenditure in this field is so small in relation to the enormous size of the disease as a worldwide problem. Perhaps, Dr. Molyneux, you want to comment upon what compels us to study a disease which is of so little risk to the developed world."

MOLYNEAUX: "There may be a lot of difficulties in doing ethically justifiable studies in the prevention and treatment of malaria. But I am quite convinced of this: that there are many of these studies that it would be unethical *not* to do. There is still a shamefully high morbidity and mortality from this disease. The mortality of cerebral malaria in a child in Africa, even with the best current therapy, is high — 37 percent in those with profound coma. Thousands of children die every month from malarial anemia. Parasites have developed at least some resistance to each of our meager range of therapeutic drugs. We must be sensitive to the needs and cultures of those most affected by malaria, but we must contribute all we can to combating this most important of all parasitic infections."

Breakthrough Sought

Scientists didn't give up the vaccine quest. Several specialists believed that in spite of the setbacks, a vaccine still offered the best chance for achieving some kind of control over the disease. At least the odds for a successful vaccine seemed greater than the odds for a viable antimalarial drug against organisms with such a formidable record in developing uncompromising resistance (Hyde, 1990).

After eradication of mosquitoes was eliminated as a method for control, there were two platforms for mounting an attack against malaria: understand the parasite or understand the disease. But the issues were not as simple as scientists once believed.

Scientists were learning to address separate endemic communities with distinctive epidemiological patterns and distinctive patterns of pathology. The patterns of symptoms were not uniform. The disease differed widely depending on the numbers of infected individuals within a community or the endemicity of the disease.

The first goal was to reduce the incidence of the disease, wrote U.S. scientist Louis Miller in 1994.[8] One proposed strategy was to develop specialized vaccines to lessen the disease in targeted locations or to prevent some of the severe disease symptoms that were apparently caused by the body's own immune response. For instance, a vaccine might be created to eliminate the characteristics of the *P. falciparum* parasite that allow it to adhere to the lining of capillaries of the victim, cutting off circulation in essential organs like the brain. It was assumed that was a cause of cerebral malaria. Miller pointed out speculations that some of the body's immune agents — or cytokines — may be contributors in the pathogenesis of cerebral malaria. But Miller recommended first that long term systematic studies of all phases of the disease were essential.

It was also believed that anemia, another grave complication of malaria, displayed differing traits in different areas. For example, in low-endemicity areas such as Thailand, the level of anemia correlated with the level of parasitemia.[9] But in Africa, parasitemia did not predict the risk of death in severely anemic children. In fact, scientists were not as certain as they used to be that anemia was only due to *P. falciparum*'s presence. Perhaps other factors contributed to the devastating anemia. Here again, there were indications of a possible role of the immune system as the cause of at least some of the symptoms (Miller, 1994).

In regions of high endemicity, the greatest suffering was borne by children under five years of age. But in areas of low endemicity, the disease affected all age groups. In highly endemic areas, although individuals over five years of age continued to harbor the parasite, the frequency of the disease was greatly reduced. That protection, known as clinical immunity, was not seen in regions with very low or only seasonal exposure to parasites.

Complications Revealed

Ordinarily, the immune system was conditioned to treat any foreign substance as an enemy. To protect the fetus, the immune system was automatically suppressed during pregnancy, leaving pregnant women in endemic areas particularly susceptible to malaria parasites and other intrusive disease agents.

Pregnant women, even those previously clinically immune, were significantly susceptible to any disease process that endangered the fetus and newborn, particularly during the mother's first pregnancy. Scientists studied the theory that malaria parasites proliferated in the placenta and also the theory that invasion of parasites into the blood cells caused low birth weight, a grave threat to babies in malarious areas. It was assumed as well that the fetus might be infected through the umbilical cord (Miller, 1994).

Another issue raised in the 1990s was the observation that malaria mortality was not much higher in communities with very high malaria transmission levels than in communities with low levels of transmission. Indeed, evidence was emerging that mortality might be lower where transmission levels were higher.

Those findings raised profoundly important concerns about the use of measures designed to reduce the malaria exposure of a population, such as impregnated bednets or transmission-blocking vaccines. Investigators have pointed out those measures could induce a short-term reduction of infection followed by a long-term increase in mortality. The reason? Some residents of a community with decreased endemicity could lose their natural immunity. A new infection could put them at risk of deadly side effects (Kwiatkowski and Marsh, 1997).

Introducing the Dendritic Cells

In another approach, a British team of scientists studied a significant way the malaria parasite may defend itself. The scientists demonstrated that the *falciparum* parasite was able to manipulate its host's immune system by inhibiting its powerful dendritic cells. To appreciate the possible implications that discovery might hold for vaccines of the future, the reader might review some of the relevant lessons of immunology.

The immune system was comprised of organs, tissues and many types of white blood cells. White cells had different sizes, shapes and functions and included the B-lymphocytes and T-lymphocytes or, simply, B-cells and T-cells.

As mentioned earlier, a normally functioning human immune system could initiate two distinct types of immune responses:

humoral and cell-mediated.[10] The humoral immunity involved the B-cells and the production of antibodies. Because antibodies couldn't attack the host's own cells, that type of immunity specifically targeted invading disease organisms that were in the human body but not inside the host's own cells. An example was a bacterial infection.

Cell-mediated immunity involved various T-cells that could directly interact with and destroy human cells infected with a virus or a parasite. That type of immunity was active against the blood stage of the malaria parasite.

Although studies of the origin and development of disease, or pathogenesis, had long focused on B-cells and T-cells, recent evidence from microbiologists placed new emphasis on the role of another kind of white blood cells, the dendritic cells, in the control of immunity. Those cells composed about one percent of all the white blood cells in the body and exerted a powerful influence over immunity. They were at least 100 times more potent than other white blood cells in inducing an immune response.

The word dendritic came from the Greek word for tree. The cells acquired that name because of their thin, scraggly, branch-like projections. They were present everywhere in the body except the brain. First visualized as Langerhans cells in the skin in 1868, their characterization began only in the last part of the 20th century. Pictures from scanning electron microscopy made dendritic cells, with all their masses of dendrites, appear like a spider web waiting for insects.

Novel Mechanism

The T-cells, often called "the warriors of the immune system," were in a dormant state when the body was attacked by foreign invaders. To do their work they needed to be awakened, and that was the role of dendritic cells.

Dendritic cells were responsible for the initial recognition of foreign invaders and for the awakening or stimulation of the T-cells from their immature state to a mature state, ready for battle. In other words, dendritic cells initiated the immune response.

The British scientists at National Blood Service in Oxford observed that intact dendretic cells exposed to red blood cells infected with *P. falciparum*, lost some of their power to stimulate the T-cells for battle. The scientists concluded, "… the maturation of dendritic cells and their subsequent ability to activate T-cells is profoundly inhibited by their interaction with intact infected erythrocytes." Erythrocytes were the human red blood cells (Urban, et al., 1999).

Those findings were significant. They indicated that *P. falciparum* possessed a novel mechanism to prevent the victim's immune system from launching a successful response against it.

The infected red blood cells had certain antigens on their surfaces that were derived from the parasite and distinguished them from uninfected red blood cells. Scientists discovered that those antigens on the surface of infected red blood cells were responsible for altering dendritic cells.

It was speculated that *P. falciparum* acquired that novel mechanism in order to disable the host's immune system early in their confrontation, when the immune response was being initiated. Thus, some scientists believed the efficacy of future vaccines might crucially depend on their capacity to stimulate and mobilize dendritic cells.

Multi-targeted Vaccines

Many scientists continued to create "multi-target" vaccines to attack the *falciparum* parasite at different stages of its development.

Dr. Altaf Lal's team at Centers for Disease Control and Prevention (CDC) in Atlanta, Georgia, was one such team working on a "multi-target" vaccine for universal use. The new vaccine was designed to make contact with the malaria parasite at every step of its life cycle in the human body. Lal said, "At each stage we're targeting several different parts" of the parasite's anatomy.

According to Lal, the experimental vaccine was designed on the principles introduced by the pioneer scientists Nussenzweig, Hoffman and Pattaroyo. The new trial vaccine, however, incorporated many more carefully selected malarial antigen epitopes[11] than were utilized in previous vaccines.

The CDC vaccine contained a total of 21 epitopes from 9 antigens from all the different stages of the parasite's life cycle. The epitopes were selected based on the *in vitro* and *in vivo* results of natural immune response studies conducted in western Kenya, and included both T-cell binding and B-cell binding epitopes (Lal, 1999).

The CDC team was optimistic about the vaccine's preliminary results in mice, and the results of testing on monkeys were expected for early 2000. According to Lal, if results continued to be encouraging, human testing would not be far off.

But some scientists still had their doubts. "One concern for an antibody-based vaccine is the selection of parasites resistant to the vaccine," Miller and Hoffman warned (Miller and Hoffman, 1998).[12] Resistant strains, in mosquitoes as well as in parasites, were proliferating.

Gene Sequencing

In another area of research, a group of insect geneticists and funding officials met in Geneva in 1999 to work on a plan to sequence the genome[13] of *Anopheles gambiae,* the large aggressive mosquito primarily responsible for spreading malaria in Africa. Scientists used the process of gene sequencing to determine the order of the DNA's chemical subunits that encoded the genetic information, ultimately associating specific traits with particular genes. With the *Anopheles,* the goal was to create a genetically modified mosquito incapable of transmitting the malaria parasite. The inspiration of the project was the fact that some strains of *Anopheles* were resistant to the parasite. They mounted an immune response that killed off the protozoan before it could mature.

Carlos Morel, director of the United Nations Special Program for Research and Training in Tropical Diseases, said, "Once we have *Anopheles* we will have all three actors in the malaria cycle" (Balter, 1999). An international team of scientists had been sequencing the genome of *Plasmodium falciparum* since 1995, and the Human Genome Project was expected to be complete before the end of year 2000.

Researchers pursuing the new project believed that a genetically modified mosquito would be the "Holy Grail" of malaria control.

Medicine from Ancient China

Meanwhile, the quest for new antimalarials continued. Military forces in particular, as well as other world travelers, still needed medicine for preventing infection and for treatment. New candidate medicines were produced from time to time that appeared to offer at least temporary protection for short-term visitors to the tropics. Typically, they were expensive, but not too expensive for the intended clientele. The parasite continued to develop resistance to just about everything drug manufacturers had to offer.

Then, in about 1975, Western chemists began hearing about the herbal medicine *qinghaosu* from Chinese literature that hailed it as a "wonder drug." But additional facts were slow to reach the U.S. and other nations of the so-called "free world." The political climate of the time and the mistrust created between East and West as a result of the "Cultural Revolution" in China made information sharing difficult. So the U.S. Military tried to find the plant growing on friendly soil. It wasn't until the 1980s that work in the U.S. on the drug could begin. Finally, in the late 1990s, with the "Cold War" thawed, the East and the West agreed to cooperate in manufacturing the drug for worldwide use (BBC Online, 1998).

Daniel L. Klayman, head of the organic chemistry section of the Division of Experimental Therapeutics at Walter Reed Army Institute of Research in Washington, D.C., was one of the Western "pioneers" who experimented with the substance. *Qinghaosu*, which was given the name artemisinin in the West, was the active compound derived from the medicinal plant *qinghao* or *Artemisia annua.* The plant was first used 2000 years ago in China for treatment of fever and refined in the last half of the 20th century by Chinese specialists. *Artemisia annua* grew wild in many places around the world — even, as Klayman found out, along the banks of the Potomac River not far from his labs.

He and his colleagues collected 60 pounds of it. He had two pots of the herb in his office when I interviewed him in 1985. The *Artemisia annua* resembled a fern, and in fact some florists used it as background in floral arrangements. Klayman and his colleagues extracted some of the drug from the plant and were able to verify the reported results from China, "at least in combating malaria in lab animals."

Klayman said artemisinin was "completely unrelated" to quinine, which was an alkaloid with a nitrogen atom and benzene rings. "Artemisinin has neither of those things. However, it does have the very unusual peroxide portion of the molecule," which he described as "remarkably stable."

"Compounds of related chemical classes can develop drug resistance," Klayman explained. "But here we have a whole new class with artemisinin, which can successfully combat malaria."

Investigations of Klayman and others into the nature of the molecule eventually led to an understanding of the mechanism of action of the drug that everyone had been waiting for.

"Artemisinin is like a bomb and there is a trigger to this bomb," according to Professor Steve Meshnick of Michigan State University, speaking at a roundtable program broadcast on BBC Radio. The molecule exploded when its peroxide portion came in contact with all that iron inside the parasite. That produced extremely toxic substances known as free radicals that killed the parasite (BBC Online, 1998).

Using a New Product

Artemisinin and its derivatives were the most potent and rapidly acting of all the antimalarial drugs developed in the late 20th century. They were 10 to 100 times more effective than other antimalarials available then in reducing the infecting malaria parasite mass. Their mode of action was to damage the parasite's membrane chemically. In addition, artemisinin and its derivatives were considered remarkably well tolerated. By the late 1990s no significant resistance to them had been reported (White, et al., 1999).

Between 1989 to 1994, a comparative study was conducted in Vietnam by a team from the medical school of Ho Chi Minh City (Hien, 1997). In fact, as of mid-1999, artemisinin had been extensively evaluated in the treatment of multiple drug-resistant *P. falciparum* in China, Myanmar, Thailand and Vietnam.

All the studies pointed to the value of the new product when used in combination with other drugs for the treatment of malaria. For example, on the northwest border of Thailand, which was believed by some people to harbor the most multi-resistant *P. falciparum* in the world, artemisinin derivatives used in combination with other drugs halted the progression of mefloquine resistance.

Although artemisinin demonstrated up to 100 percent capacity in clearing malaria parasites, it was established that the drug and its derivatives had an unacceptably high recrudescence rate, less than seven days, when used as the only mode of treatment. Consequently, experts from various countries decided against using artemisinin or its derivatives alone. They chose instead to reserve the drug for use in combination with other antimalarials.

Caution in Drug Use

The strategy for combining drugs with independent modes of action to retard the emergence of resistance was first developed in antituberculosis chemotherapy. The strategy was later adopted for cancer chemotherapy and also for the treatment of AIDS.

In the case of the new malaria medicine, there were two major advantages in using it with another appropriate drug. First, the scientists figured that, since resistance arose from mutations, the chance for simultaneous emergence of resistance to two medicines seemed minimal. In addition, a rapidly acting drug like artemisinin and a slowly eliminated drug such as mefloquine could complement the actions of one another rather nicely.

For example, trials in Thailand showed that a 3-day treatment with artemisinin or its derivatives rapidly eliminated most of the infection. Then the remaining parasites (as little as 0.000001 percent of the original mass) were exposed to high concentrations of slowly eliminated mefloquine alone to prevent recurrence (White, et al., 1999).

Views about the widespread use of artemisinin were not unanimous. Some specialists believed that artemisinin was so effective for treating severe malaria that it should be conserved. It was recommended that it be saved for use only in areas with a special, urgent need. Such restraint might protect the drug from selecting resistant strains.

Other experts proposed that artemisinin be used only in combination with other drugs. That way the risk of development of drug-resistant strains would be satisfactorily reduced, those specialists believed.

The experts did not know if or when artemisinin would join the long list of drugs to which the parasite had developed resistance. However, artemisinin advocates stressed that just an extra five or 10 years of efficacy could be incredibly valuable in areas in Africa where, as Oxford scientist Kevin Marsh reported, "a health calamity looms within the next few years" (*Ibid.*).

Price Tag

Scientists were becoming outspoken about a delicate but critical topic: the faltering enthusiasm of some of the traditional supporters of malaria research. Pharmaceutical companies usually eager for a role in the creation of a cure for the world's worst disease were having doubts. Those doubts were discussed at a symposium called "Malaria: Waiting for the Vaccine," hosted by the London School of Hygiene and Tropical Medicine in 1991.[14]

Some participants believed malaria experts should learn more about practical economics of vaccine research. Plans were proposed for integration of cost data with epidemiological data.

Malariologist Chev Kidson reflected on some of the highlights of the symposium in a special report.[15] He wrote, "Perhaps now is the time to begin putting fiscal clothing on this skeleton by way of economic modeling which encompasses the molecular and epidemiological databases to build dynamic concepts of what is affordable alongside what will work" (Kidson, 1991).[16] Critical questions were: How much were the scientists spending on creating the vaccines? How many sick people were likely to benefit? When can one conclude that a given project was actually cost-effective?

Kidson said the "hype" over malaria research "bred the unreal expectations and led to the pessimism" that was heard in many quarters. But he said that, with time, support and quieter opportunity, "there is reason to believe that a number of vaccines on the drawing boards would give some protection to at least some target groups" (*Ibid.*).

At the same time, private industry was not expected to keep sinking large sums in projects with scant expectations of profit. Kidson pointed out that the development cost of medical research often was "written off" or absorbed by commercial interests, but not production costs. "Industry has to make money to prosper," he said.

Kidson also raised the theme that was heard more and more frequently in the post-DDT period. Malaria research and planning should be developed in collaboration with people from the communities with an intimate knowledge of local history and conditions.

As the years passed, more specialists identified obstacles to successful vaccine production. Louis Miller and Steve Hoffman said, "The main obstacle to vaccine development has been the absence of industrial interest in blood stage vaccines because they do not expect profits that would warrant the investment." Many of the parasite's blood stage antigens had been identified as effective in vaccinating mice and monkeys, but few of the antigens were tested in human subjects. Human trials were too expensive for most research organizations (Miller and Hoffman, 1998).

Also, some experts pointed out that areas where malaria was endemic generally had poor infrastructure for health surveillance. A valid malaria vaccine trial was a major undertaking (Kwiatkowski, 1997).

Meanwhile, more people were dying, and the poor were getting poorer.

Competition For Funding

The obligation of a community to take care of its poor and needy members was probably almost as old as humankind. The obligation was felt acutely in Europe in the 19th century when the scope of health needs in its tropical colonies was recognized and when the industrial revolution attracted poor people from the countryside to the congested and unhygienic big cities. The enormous number of casualties from World Wars I and II added to the dimension of suffering that could not be ignored by compassionate governments, particularly if the governments wanted to stay in power. Sweeping reforms were introduced.

Other forces, meanwhile, were competing for health budgets.

Breakthroughs in health sciences in the 1930s and 1940s drew public attention and money away from public health projects. It was popularly believed that modern science would exert such mastery over disease that public health care, or preventive care, would become expendable.

Subsequent years shattered that hubris. Laboratory creations seemed helpless, for instance, against hunger, poverty, and the mosquito "carrying death in its spittle" (Russell, 1943).

Promise of Alma-Ata

By the 1960s or the 1970s, as scientific solutions for malaria and other grave threats had proved unreliable and health and living standards in poor countries disintegrated, international health authorities searched for new ways the rich countries of the world might collaborate to help the poor. International health conferences and forums looked for collaborative solutions for extending health care to the developing world. Halfdan Mahler, who became director general of WHO in 1973, led the quest.

The result was a unique international health convention in 1978 held in Alma-Ata,[17] in the former Soviet Central Asia. The meeting was called by the World Health Organization and UNICEF (United Nations International Children's Emergency Fund), and the venue was provided by the former Soviet Union, which at the time was strongly committed to universal primary health care. The conference was held under the chairmanship of B.V. Petrovsky, Minister of Health of the Soviet Union.

The International Conference on Primary Health Care, with representatives of 134 sovereign nations in attendance, was popularly called Alma-Ata. The focus on health equity and social justice between and within nations gave a strong impetus to primary health care programs for neglected communities and neglected problems throughout the developing world, including the accelerating problem of malaria. The final report of Alma-Ata rendered the issues deceptively clear, inspiring and at the same time undeniable:

> *Primary Health Care is essential health care made univer-*
> *sally accessible to individuals and families in the community by*
> *means acceptable to them, through their full participation and at*
> *a cost that the community and country can afford. It forms an*
> *integral part both of the country's health system of which it is the*
> *nucleus and of the overall social and economic development of*
> *the community.*

The Alma-Ata meeting closed with a promise of "Health for All, by the year 2000." The promise sounded great but was unattainable.

World Health Strategies

Alma-Ata was a working meeting with serious practical discussions of specific problems and options for addressing them. According to one participant, the meeting "reflected a deep desire to counteract the fatalist feeling that long-term political socio-economic trends were bringing the world closer and closer to the danger of self-destruction, whether from universal warfare, the escalation of 'conventional wars' or from the slow but inexorable distractions of the world's ecological balance." The achievement was hailed as a "major turning point in the development of health care throughout the world" (Venediktov, 1998). In other words, Alma-Ata made everyone feel good, at least for a while. The deadline of year 2000 seemed a long way off. Participants assumed that 22 years would certainly allow enough time to reach the group's goals.

The first 10 years of the challenge of "Health for All" were active. Beginning almost immediately, the planners unveiled a policy they called Selective Primary Health Care, or SPHC. Basically, it meant attacking one disease at a time. The selection of each disease, or specific health problem, was based largely on

196

the anticipation of generous public and private funding, and large donors preferred to support health initiatives with a publicly defined beginning and end. Several separate campaigns sponsored by a variety of interests were launched, including childhood immunizations, planned parenthood, oral rehydration instruction to save children with diarrhea, AIDS, TB and more. A typical campaign for humanitarian aid was launched amid fanfare spotlighting well-known movie stars, musicians and sports celebrities.

What the campaigns lacked was effective coordination with community health providers from participating countries. The plans also lacked epidemiological studies showing status of disease at each location. Each campaign was designed and executed with the assumptions that the needs and sensitivities of each community were the same; that the disease displayed the same characteristics each place.

Each campaign was grounded in a technology that permitted a system for tabulating how many people would be protected from infection. That is, how many lives would be saved — in theory. Thus sponsors could convert that figure to a prevention rate that might be useful in future promotions (Chen, 1988; Gish, 1992; Yach, 1996).

Reactions From the Experts

One of the early critics of the new SHPC strategies was a prominent physician from India, a specialist in primary health care in poor rural areas. He was Debabar Banerji.[18] He didn't mince his words. He said the new policies violated the ideals and promises of Alma-Ata. He called the policies "astonishingly defective in concept, design and implementation." Banerji was particularly critical of what he saw as indifference to the special needs and customs of specific local communities.

The health establishment in India, like other places with a bitter history of colonialism and internal fighting, had been a critical plank in rallying poor folks to the independence struggle. According to Banerji, the new country owed its political survival to its health services. As Banerji said, "After Independence, India's ruling class, which had led the freedom struggle against the colonial rulers, was impelled by the working class to fulfill the promises it had made while mobilizing them for the struggle. This was the compelling motive force for its ushering in very ambitious health programs to cover the needs of the unserved and the underserved during the first two decades of independence, even though the country faced massive problems."

Banerji said, "The long experience of India in developing its health services has escaped the attention of scholars from rich countries." He added that universal campaigns introduced from the outside were sometimes resented (Banerji, 1999).

Nigeria's Experience

Local physicians and authorities in some other areas as well did not appreciate the "campaign" style of distributing health care. One critic was retired Nigerian Minister of Health, Olikoye Ransome-Kuti. He said the visiting health teams from donor agencies typically provided everything needed to accomplish the task assigned. "The tools are there. It's just that we don't get them to people in a way that is effective to reduce mortality and morbidity," he said.[19]

Rehydration Therapy

Another problematic campaign was the well-publicized drive to teach mothers how to rehydrate their children who might be in danger of dying from dehydration following a bad case of diarrhea. The instruction was the same everywhere. A health worker from the outside introduced sachets of salts and sugars to be mixed with water to protect the child. The mothers were told to use that product and nothing else for restoring water to the child's body.

What was missing from that picture? Plenty. The worker from the outside usually was unaware of the pathology causing the diarrhea. For instance: Did the people have access to pure water? Did each family have a system for washing their vegetables, dishes, and hands? Did the mothers already have materials available locally to rehydrate their children? Dependence on a product imported from the outside could be counter-productive.

In at least one village, mothers stopped their traditional treatments when the sachets were not delivered on schedule. In that situation it was possible that more infants actually were harmed than were helped by rehydration campaigns.

Local health authorities became wary of SPHC campaigns. AIDS campaigns and the TB campaign also were criticized: AIDS, because the campaigns seldom addressed the issues in a culturally acceptable way; and TB, because it was not considered a problem requiring special attention from outside experts.

Some campaigns apparently were organized to respond to special interests of the sponsors. For instance, in the 1980s, four countries were identified as good potential market areas, anticipating the looming economic boom. Those places were targeted for public health programs that might enhance their ability to function in a market economy.

Occasionally a SPHC program expanded to empower an entire community to adopt new systems to effect long-lasting improvements in the development of the community at large. The Rockefeller Foundation cited four locations where that happened. They were Sri Lanka, China, Costa Rica and the Indian state of Kerala (Halstead, et al., 1987).

Deadline Approaches

As year 2000 drew near, more criticism arose, not criticism of the Alma-Ata goals but of the process. One WHO official noted that "the widening gap between rich and poor population groups and countries presents a formidable obstacle for attempts to reduce inequalities in health status" (Yach, 1996). In his article in the World Health Forum (V. 17; 1996), Yach invited other international health professionals to comment about whether the Alma-Ata follow-up goals should be abandoned, altered, or continued as begun.[20]

He said, "New obstacles have arisen to challenge continuing progress, some gains are not being maintained and in most parts of the world there is evidence of increased inequality." Yach said there was "an increasing preoccupation with making health systems more efficient technically and economically" but not necessarily more responsive to the needs of the community.

A common theme among the answers submitted to Yach was the need to create stronger links with the communities being served. One responder pointed out that the per capita health budget in many developing countries was less than U.S. $10 per year. He said, "A process needs to occur that would place emphasis on the health of populations rather than the disease of individuals. Until scarce health resources are allocated according to population-based disease prevention and health promotion priorities, health for all will continue to be an elusive goal"[21] (Spencer, 1996).

Health and Development

Mozambique, a poor African country burdened by a legacy of war and a huge debt to foreign banks, had a historic commitment to provide health care for its citizenry. Like many countries in the developing world, Mozambique's emergence was linked to the ambitions of imperial powers.

In 1497, Vasco da Gama rounded South Africa's Cape of Good Hope and set his sails north into the Indian Ocean in search of a convenient route to the fabled cities of Asia. The Portuguese explorer sailed into Quelimane harbor at the mouth of the northernmost tributary of the great Zambezi River, which linked the highlands and lakes region of southeastern Africa with the Indian Ocean. The banks of the river and sheltered coves on the ocean had been settled by African agriculturists joined by Arabs who established so-called Zenj city-states and traded with merchants from Arab countries to the north and India to the east. The Arabs dealt with a variety of valuable products over the years including cotton, food products, and Africans captured for slavery. The slave trade lasted until the middle of the 19th century (Encyclopedia Britannica, 1965). Reports said the settlers made "great progress" combating malaria that was concentrated near breeding grounds of mosquitoes in the lowlands in early days (*Ibid.*).

By 1513, Portuguese settlers had ascended the Zambezi, establishing trading posts over 1,600 miles of the coastline (Langer, 1980; Encarta Encyclopedia Online, 2000).

Later sporadic native uprisings against foreign intruders were a problem in Mozambique, which was not as prosperous as the colonies owned by other European empires, Britain and Germany, that colonized the region. In 1895, those two countries gave Mozambique a joint loan to finance its maintenance. Then, in 1907, the Mozambican government established a legislative council representing European interests. Portugal granted some autonomy to local interests and designated Mozambique as an overseas province of Portugal in 1951 (Encyclopedia Britannica, 1965; Langer, 1980).

Agitation continued to build among Mozambique's black population, joined by members of the independence movement, Frelimo. An open revolt against Portuguese rule started in 1964. Eleven years later, in 1975, Portugal was crippled by its own political turmoil and granted Mozambique independence (Encarta Encyclopedia Online, 2000). But peace didn't last long and a civil war was on the way.

Mozambique's leaders closed their borders with the Rhodesian regime and supported the Zimbabweans in their struggle for independence. "As a result, Ian Smith's Rhodesia and later South Africa intervened to pursue their own interests by creating and sustaining a rebel movement, Renamo," according to Colin Legum.[22]

The independent state of Mozambique was quick to address its obligations to provide public health facilities. According to a U.S. specialist in international public health, Dr. Steve Gloyd, the services provided were considered "models for other developing countries" (Gloyd, 1996).

Writing in 1996, Gloyd characterized the health issues. He said, "The new government focused on prevention, making essential drugs available, and improving access to basic health care. By 1978, three years after winning independence, nearly 100 percent of the population had been immunized, and four years later more than 1,200 health posts had been constructed. More than 8,000 mid-level health workers had been trained and placed in service" (*Ibid.*).

"The top echelons were well-trained and had substantial experience in public health, but little management training. Mid-level health workers then usually had two to three years of specialized training. Virtually all of that development was carried out by the government, which was spending about 11 percent of its budget on health" (*Ibid.*).

According to Gloyd, most of the projects were locally managed. Very few non-governmental organizations (NGOs) worked in Mozambique in those days.

Mozambique's 16-year civil war nearly destroyed the country. Although Mozambique triumphed in the end, costs to repair the destruction to the country's infrastructure in the fighting were more than the government could handle. The health and resettlement costs alone were huge. By the end of the 20th century, the U.S. had spent about $25 million in Mozambique to deactivate mines left over from the civil war.[23] About 1.5 million people became refugees, and 700,000 civilians and combatants were killed. According to Gloyd, by 1988, 600 health posts had been destroyed, and economic development was paralyzed outside major cities.

202

Rebuilding Mozambique's health services was difficult and expensive. International agencies and affluent countries in the developed world loaned money for recovery. As was the custom in financing development projects, lenders imposed restraints on the debtor country. Like in most countries in Africa, Mozambique's economy was placed on a structural adjustment policy, or SAP. The country was required to realign its economic priorities, abandoning its emphasis on health and education and redirecting resources to an invigorated private sector. From the lenders' perspective, the best course of development was to stimulate the output of products for export. Then the debtors would have a better chance to afford interest payments and qualify for new loans.

It sounded logical. But Mozambique was one of only a few African countries able to meet its SAP. The terms were rigid.

Mozambique's SAP required that its health care budget be cut to 2 percent of the national budget, down from 11 percent. "That meant the country had to charge 15 times more for health care services than in the past," said Gloyd. Many NGOs assigned health workers to Mozambique to improve service, but that, according to Gloyd, often made matters worse.

Gloyd described conditions in Manica Province on the border with Zimbabwe, where he worked as an advisor to the government. He said, "Health workers from the outside came with large budgets, well-equipped offices, fleets of cars and trucks, affluent housing expectations, and generous salaries. Indeed, many of the 20 NGOs in Manica Province had budgets larger than what the whole province could spend on health. Staff salaries were typically two to 100 times higher than those of their Mozambican counterparts, many of whom had similar or higher levels of training. The Manica Province director of community health programs coordinated activities of several NGOs whose drivers and cleaning staff earned two or three times more than he did."

Morale among the local staff was bad, negatively affecting health care delivery. Gloyd said the presence and well-meaning activities of the outsiders, "engendered inefficiency, duplications, resentment and dependence." Gloyd was confident, however, that management adjustments might eventually diminish the frustration created by the NGOs, especially if the visiting personnel were offered more participation in joint planning, management and evaluation of programs.

Meanwhile, Mozambique was earning a good, although painful, record for paying interest on old loans. By the late 1990s, when some lenders were responding to outside pressure to grant relief to their borrowers, Mozambique was lobbying for special consideration.

The government was already paying 10 times more for servicing old debts than it paid for health care. President Joachim Chissano appealed for special terms considering the huge cost to repair damage done to its infrastructure during its civil war. The president also brought up another issue. He protested the high servicing fees imposed on Mozambique. He cited the reconstruction loans granted Germany after its defeat in World War II. Germany paid 3.5 percent for servicing its development debt, whereas Mozambique was paying 20 percent for its debt (BBC Online, 1999). Eventually, several international lenders were pledging debt relief for the poorest countries of the world. But details had not been resolved by the end of the 20th century.

Interest Payment

By the 1970s and 1980s, a growing number of newly independent African governments were in need of development loans from international lenders. By the 1990s, many of the countries were having trouble keeping up with the interest payments. New jargon was born. The heavily indebted poor countries were called HIPCs. And the recovery plans to help HIPCs and other developing countries regain their financial credibility were called structural adjustment policies, or as mentioned before, SAPs.

By the late 1990s, 29 African governments had signed up for SAPs with the World Bank. A UN Development Programme (UNDP) report said that, by the end of the millennium the combined debts owed by the poorest 41 countries was $212 billion, up from $183 billion in 1990 and $55 billion in 1980 (BBC Online, 1999). As it happened in Mozambique, health care throughout Africa was jeopardized.

Another UNDP report in 1997 maintained that if African governments were relieved of their debt obligations the funds could be used to save the lives of millions of children by the year 2000.

Most of the SAPs the highly indebted countries were placed on, however, required the recipients to cut back health and social services in favor of income generating projects like produce for export. At a meeting in September, 1996, the World Bank and the International Monetary Fund identified more than 40 HIPCs that needed help in reducing their debt burdens to tolerable levels. But help often required new loans and restrictions on ways the new money could be spent. Health care was not a high priority for international lenders. There was no tangible profit.

Mozambique was one of the first few African countries designated by the World Bank and the International Monetary Fund for complicated debt adjustment programs granting extensions of interest payments but imposing intricate terms specifying how the new money would be used.

In addition to cutting back health services, Mozambique was required to impose a value-added tax (VAT) on merchandise, an imposition widely opposed. The Mozambican government protested both the new conditions. President Chissano protested that the limited debt relief was insufficient. He claimed his country was entitled to special consideration because of the destruction and suffering inflicted by the forces of apartheid South Africa during the civil war that followed his country's independence. (He was not the only African leader to ask for debt relief for reconstruction following assault from outside forces.)

Alternative Approaches

Meanwhile, during the last decade of the century, support was building for more comprehensive debt forgiveness with no strings attached. An international coalition called Jubilee 2000 was joined by influential scholars, church leaders and activists from entertainment and sports organizations in Europe and North America with many activists in Asia and Latin America. Its goal was total debt forgiveness for highly indebted countries. One of the group's conferences in Washington, D.C. in September 1999 focused on "Alternative Approaches to Debt Relief." Co-sponsors were The Global Coalition for Africa (GCA) and the Center for International Development, Harvard University (CID). Attendees included officials from highly indebted African countries, the African Development Bank and the UN Development Program.

Several speakers drew attention to the need to include representatives from the HIPCs in planning sessions. They specifically urged that special consideration be given to the emergency needs of "post-conflict countries" where large amounts of money were needed to repair damage to sanitation facilities, housing and infrastructure.

The well-organized and well-publicized appeals of Jubilee 2000 were effective. Several informed observers gave the group credit for developments that followed. The German government announced it would relieve all its poor third world debtors of obligations to repay. Then, at a summit meeting in June, 1999, in Cologne, Germany and other countries in the Group of seven leading industrialized nations, or G-7, produced a document called the Cologne Initiative. Members were encouraged to consider strategies for third world debt cancellation.

In September, 1999, Pope John Paul II issued a letter supporting Jubilee 2000, stating that the jubilee was the time when the entire community was called on to restore human relations. In Washington in the same month, President Clinton pledged to initiate forgiveness of 100 percent of the money owed to U.S. lenders by poor countries of sub-Saharan Africa (Sanger, 1999). Later the U.S. Congress approved the proposal, without any restrictions on how the new funds should be spent by recipient countries (BBC Online, 1999).

Canada also joined the campaign for debt relief for poor countries. In December, 1999, it cancelled the entire debt burden of $600,000 owed by Bangladesh. Canada's Minister for International Cooperation, Maria Minna, said the action was taken because of Bangladesh's record of timely payments on the debt in spite of the devastating floods it had endured.

The movement did have its critics. Certain countries where the population was most impoverished, were countries richly endowed with natural resources like diamonds, gold and oil. Often those same countries were ruled by elite families who diverted the rich natural resources for their own extravagant use like mansions on the Riviera. Some of the riches were used to wage war on neighbors or to engage security forces for personal protection.

Several international lenders opposed any debt relief. Some observers just didn't agree with the strategies of Jubilee 2000. The London Times called the plan "a senselessly impulsive gesture," adding "it could only provide a tantalizingly short-term sense of progress" (BBC Online, 1999).

Another emphatic opponent of debt relief was the U.K. Centre for Accountability and Debt Relief (CADRE). It offered a specific plan to correct the problems. The director, Karl Ziegler, said advocates for debt relief like Jubilee 2000 attracted well-meaning supporters based on intellectually dishonest arguments. As quoted by BBC News, he said, "It is not debt that starves children, but corruption" (*Ibid.*).

Ziegler's organization recommended assignment of auditors to each debtor country to oversee the allocation of funds and to suggest corrections where needed. He described an early program that was under examination. The U.K. Chancellor recommended that auditors be installed in the new Nigerian government's Central Bank, a state-owned oil company and the Ministry of Finance. Such a program, he said, would benefit over-borrowed nations, the world's poor people, and "the Jubilee 2000 campaign would finally be put on the right track.".

Some of the most damning criticisms came from experts most knowledgeable about international debt issues. An OXFAM study showed that the SAP strategies actually led to unemployment in Africa. The report said "The reality of SAPs is that they have locked Africa into a downward spiral of disinvestment and low growth, all in the familiar name of defeating inflation" (Legum, 1999).

World Bank President James Wolfenson accepted what the critics had said all along. He said, "One thing which has been learnt in recent years is an absolute recognition that, unless you have sound social policies, you cannot have sound economic policies. That is crystal clear. Unless you have a solid base with the people, unless you are concerned with the rights of the individual, unless you are concerned with elements of social responsibility and social justice, you cannot have peace and you cannot have safe investing" (*Ibid.*).

The Author Must Wonder…

In the year 2000, the author must wonder how many more centuries malaria would be around, humbling humankind, riding in the spittle of a mosquito?

The author must also wonder what else she can do to help illuminate malaria's puzzle for the general reader. Perhaps she can show the reader communities where malaria has taken the greatest toll.

[1] Influential American malariologist and writer, active in the US and abroad from the 1920s to the 1950s.

[2] The dialogue was printed in *Journal of Medical Ethics*, 1992, 18: 189-192. Reprinted with permission from the BMJ Publishing Group.

[3] The Nuremberg code for research on human subjects was established in 1949 in response to mistreatment of human subjects in Nazi Germany. The Helsinki declaration, adopted in 1964 and revised in 1975, was a recommendation for conduct of clinical research.

[4] Ajayi O. O. "Taboos and clinical research in West Africa," *Journal of Medical Ethics* 1980; 6: 61-63.

[5] "Most importantly, do no harm."

[6] See table on pg. 125 for detailed definition.

[7] The condition or quality of causing malformations of an embryo or fetus.

[8] His expansive report 'Malaria Pathogenesis' in *Science*, 24 June 1994, was co-authored by M.F. Good of Brisbane, Australia, and G. Milon of Paris.

[9] A condition where parasites are present in the blood.

[10] See 'The role of the immune system' on pg. 112 for more details.

[11] Also known as antigenic determinants, these are exposed active areas of the antigen molecule with which an antibody can combine. Most complex molecules contain numerous epitopes.

[12] Louis H. Miller at National Institute of Health, and Stephen L. Hoffman of the Naval Medical Research Institute.

[13] The entire genetic content.

[14] Other sponsors of the symposium were Overseas Development Administration, Swiss Tropical Institute, WHO, and the World Bank.

[15] Member of the Faculty of Tropical Medicine, Mahidol University, Bangkok.

[16] Responding to presentations by Anne Mills and Somkid Kaewsonthi at "Malaria: Waiting for the Vaccine" symposium.

[17] Capital of the Republic of Kazakhstan until late in the 20th Century. Renamed Almaty. Was considered one of the most beautiful cities of the former USSR.

[18] Professor, Centre of Social Medicine and Community Health. Jawaharlal Nehru University, New Delhi. Publications include a 16-year study in 19 villages of the relationships between health technology and people.

[19] See 'Rural health infrastructure' on pg. 230 for more details.

[20] Derek Yach, Chief of the Policy Action Coordination Team, Division of Development of Policy, Programme and Evaluation, World Health Organization

[21] Harrison C. Spencer, Dean of the London School of Hygiene and Tropical Medicine.

[22] Colin Legum, a prominent political activist and scholar, was banned from his homeland of South Africa for many years under the Apartheid regime. He returned to his home in Cape Town when the new South African government was installed.

[23] The U.S. also set aside $2.5 million in March 2000 to assist Mozambique with land mines that had been dislodged by floods a month earlier.

PART III
Malaria in the Developing World

This is an issue of vision.
We have been looking at malaria with the vision of an outsider.
Now we'll turn our vision to places where malaria is deeply
embedded in the culture, environment and hopes of the people.

Chapter 9
Sub-Saharan Africa

IN THE EVENING, the heat of the day did not dissipate. It merely seemed to shift a little as the harmattan wind carried in a film of sand from the Sahara on its way to the Atlantic coast. The sand was not always visible, but it wiped out the sky. I was aware of the harmattan by the strange rosy cast near the horizon and by the gritty taste in my mouth.

An African physician escorted me through the streets and alleys of the old market of Ibadan, Nigeria, identifying the small shady pools typical of those where mosquito larvae might be found. One pool was in a stopped-up gully beside the folding table of a vendor. Her baby, with a traditional charm around her neck to protect her from disease, was asleep on a piece of cardboard in the shade of the table, her bare arm close to the water. The doctor said, "Now you see where malaria is being transmitted."

Africa was overwhelmingly ridden with malaria. An estimated one million or more African babies died every year from the disease. The continent accounted for an estimated 90 percent of the malaria infections in the world and 80 percent of the active cases (White, et al., 1999). Most of it was caused by *Plasmodium falciparum*, the deadly species.

View From the Alley

An alley behind us vibrated as an opulently dressed wedding party swaggered by, followed by drummers and trumpeters. We passed stalls displaying an assortment of traditional cures, including various charms and high stacks of bark and dried plants for medicinal teas. Traditional products were widely used for malaria, even among African professionals who had studied abroad. One prominent Ibadan lawyer said she no longer bought "Western" medicine for malaria. The traditional medicine worked just as well, she said. At least it offered some relief from the fever and pain, and she could afford the price.

On a hilltop on one side of the old town, the research director of the Nigerian Forestry Service made his own personal malaria medicine. He told us he compiled lists of ingredients of various medicines offered by traditional practitioners, chose the substances he thought might be active against malaria parasites and combined them himself. He drank his own mixture in a tea whenever he felt he was coming down with the disease.

Like many other people in Africa, he believed that having something handy at home for self treatment saved him from the full force of the disease. Many Africans told me they were aware of the disease before the symptoms struck. They spoke of a distinctive but difficult-to-describe prodromal feeling that gave a warning. That sounded logical; hundreds of thousands of parasites had been infecting the body before the fever and pain were felt.

New Garbage Trucks

Driving back to the University of Ibadan College of Medicine, we saw a fleet of bright new yellow garbage trucks parked by the river. They had been donated by the government of Japan. The scene reminded me of the mahouts of Sri Lanka washing their elephants in a shallow river. I was reminded also of a conversation I had with a malaria specialist in Zambia. I had asked, "What would you choose, if you could have anything you wanted to control malaria?" The answer: "Garbage trucks." I hoped Zambia got some new garbage trucks too.

At the college campus, my escort pointed out the many ornamental trees in the mall that were disfigured by bare patches on the trunks. He said a student may cut a piece of any bark that looked promising and chew it or save it for tea, hoping to gain some protection from malaria. Many students had identified individual trees as personal favorites.

The Yoruba people from Ibadan and nearby regions of western Nigeria had a rich tradition of herbal medicine, once driven underground by the old colonial government from Britain and later supported by the country's national leaders. Government laboratories had been testing some of the traditional substances with no immediate reports of finding curative properties in any of them. Several medicinal plants, however, showed some efficacy in terms of symptom control. The search for a natural cure and the faith in materials found locally and used for generations continued into modern times.

An estimated 30 to 50 percent of medicines consumed worldwide were traditional medicines made from natural substances. Throughout history, areas where malaria was endemic had particularly rich traditions of local cures. And of course, Nigeria was one of those areas.

Search for New Medicines

In 1989, Nigeria's Ministry of Health published guidelines for malaria control. The writers acknowledged a partial reliance of large segments of the population on traditional medicines for

215

symptom control. One substance selected for further research was Dogonyaro (*Azadirhacta indica*), cited as a widely recognized antimalarial plant. The publication said the aqueous or watery extract of the leaves was demonstrated to have "antimalarial activity" (Federal Ministry of Health, Nigeria, 1989). Meanwhile studies were continuing to isolate the antimalarial components of the plant family of Simaroubacceae, well known in Nigeria and elsewhere for curative properties (Ajaiyeoba, et al., 1999).

The government publication also reviewed guidelines for malaria treatment and control, including several provisions for practical community protection. The Ministry report stressed the need for community-based prevention and control operations as opposed to chemoprophylatic strategies. At the top of the list were environmental modifications, including installation of irrigation systems, closing water holes, altering water levels, changing water salinity and deforestation. Personal protection measures were mentioned as well, including the promotion of mosquito nets, insect repellents, window screens, clothing protection, and placement of human settlement away from mosquito breeding areas. In addition, recommendations were made for biological control, like the introduction of predatory bacteria, fish, fungi and other biologic agents (Federal Ministry of Health, Nigeria, 1989).

More recently, a team of Nigerian doctors at the Department of Pharmacology and Therapeutics of the University of Ibadan's Postgraduate Institute of Medical Research and Training began research on the curative effects of the Chinese herbal derivative, artemether, in children infected with falciparum malaria (Sowunmi & Oduola, 1996).

Also, a group of Nigerian researchers writing in 1992 identified separate attitudes among different folks about the disease. For example, men and women had different views about malaria. Although the women correctly identified the cause of malaria according to the report, "the men and the traditional healers said malaria was caused by such things as staying in the sun too long, bad water and indiscriminate sex. Thus, the preventive measures they adopted were often inappropriate" (Okonofua, et al., 1992).

The team recognized traditional medicine's role in symptom control but stressed the fact that a lack of scientific knowledge of the disease's etiology — or cause — could hinder the effectiveness of traditional therapies and treatments *(Ibid.).*

Whether due to the cost or inefficacy of Western medicines or the weakness of traditional ones, about 40 new patients entered the University Hospital with malaria each day, and they were usually very, very ill. The death toll of malaria throughout the country had been rising.

Perspectives on Prevention

Many Western scientists wanted to expand research for creation of new malaria medicines. But not all Africans believed an array of new medicines was going to control malaria. Excessive international emphasis was placed on advanced medical technology, according to Awash Teklehaimanot, an Ethiopian doctor on the staff of WHO in Geneva. Teklehaimanot was a member of the Committee for the Study on Malaria Prevention and Control, a 19-member international panel assembled by the Institute of Medicine of the National Academy of Sciences in Washington, D.C. The panel was gathering recommendations for new U.S. government funding for malaria research, prevention and control. Teklehaimanot's criticisms, as well as the panel's suggestions, appeared in the book *"Malaria, Obstacles and Opportunities"* published by the Academy in 1991.

"The deteriorating malaria situation," he said, "must not be seen as a justification for undertaking more research." Money would be better spent, according to Teklehaimanot, in training health workers in the countries most severely stricken and in helping those countries to strengthen and broaden their health infrastructures to reach all communities, no matter how remote.

He recommended that malaria control be incorporated

217

within the overall community health care structure of each country. He recommended as well that teachers receive training to help children and parents understand the way the malaria parasites functioned, the role of the mosquito and the ways communities and families could prevent the disease, or reduce its transmission. There was a lot that local folks might do for themselves, after they understood how the disease was transmitted, the Ethiopian doctor said.

One illustration of that theme was related to me in Africa by a friend and father of five small children. He said people in his family compound were always getting malaria. They were suffering more than any other family in their community, and he couldn't figure out why. Then, searching the yards around his home, he discovered the problem. Barrels of palm oil his father produced were left by the roadside for pickup. About two inches of rainwater had collected on top of each barrel where mosquito larvae were breeding. He said, "We were producing malaria as well as palm oil." He rolled the barrels over on their sides, and the family practically never got malaria again.

Historic Obstacles

The history of Ibadan fascinated me. In its early history, it was a crossroads attracting migrations of outsiders who brought with them disease organisms from far away, including malaria that thrived wherever populations mingled. Early traders established overland routes from across the Sahara. A mixture of strains of malaria was also brought in by clans of Yoruba tribal people waging a series of wars back and forth across the region.

Periodically, refugees from a multitude of civil wars moved to the nearby hills that eventually became the city of Ibadan. The British colonialists, merchants, missionaries, explorers and sailors who came to West Africa had high infection and death rates from malaria, and the area came to be called the "White Man's Grave."

In 1900, the British governor of Nigeria, a physician himself, conducted a massive malaria control program in the nearby capital of Lagos, which was built on a marsh. He dispatched uniformed health inspectors called "woolie woolies" throughout the neighborhoods to make certain each house owner was keeping his or her property clear of still waters where mosquitoes might breed. If the inspector found undrained or uncovered water on the person's land, the owner might be fined or sent to jail. In addition, the governor organized groups of African women to give away quinine to schoolchildren.

Those strategies didn't work, but not because they were ill conceived. Historians concluded that the governor, weakened from multiple malarial attacks himself, was simply ahead of his time and had to abandon his program prematurely. His project was described as "an idealism that certainly reached too high for that day."

Over the years, history showed that sanitation projects to prevent mosquitoes from breeding close to human habitation could help control the disease, even in the tropics.

The Tides of Colonialism

One Nigerian scientist said the burden of malaria in his country convinced the British government to give up its plans for a large permanent settlement in Nigeria. The British government changed its colonial immigration policy and turned its attention from Nigeria to South Africa. British imperialists faced belligerent opposition in South Africa from the native black tribes and the Boers who where there already. But malaria was not so bad there.

As of the early 1990s, no independent Nigerian government had undertaken large-scale antimalaria projects for community sanitation, surveillance and health education. It was thought that such activities would remind the local inhabitants of their erstwhile colonial rulers. One Nigerian man told me, "People here don't want anybody from the outside interfering with their communities," and for many Nigerians, government authorities were considered "outsiders." In a country with volatile politics and bitter memories, leaders were cautious about "interfering." One local doctor, for example, said that when he went to a village to survey the status of malaria, people were suspicious. He said he had to take care first to convince the chief that he did not represent the government. Then, and only then, could the doctor start to examine patients.

No Place Like Home

By the end of the 20th century Africa, the "cradle of malaria," was still the continent where malaria seemed most at home. Historians offered several reasons: the continent's sweltering heat, the presence of the super vector *An. gambiae*, the emergence of drug-resistant parasites and the pervasive poverty. But many people believed the real reason for malaria's success in Africa was the lack of health infrastructure, particularly the infrastructure serving rural areas or interests.

Also, by the end of the 20th century, only a few African communities were free of endemic malaria. Those were mostly former European colonies that had to fight their oppressors to gain political independence or countries shattered by internal wars fought to address old territorial disputes. The ravaged regions were left without even the basic requirements for community health delivery. They had virtually no rural infrastructure adequate for protection from infectious diseases and no system for food distribution to prevent malnutrition.

Those countries still were mired in chronic political upheavals that deprived their citizenry of even the most basic disease protection. Partly due to the legacy of the Cold War, many of those fledgling governments were spending far more than they could afford on armaments and the military, at the expense of funding for social programs like education, nutrition, small business development, land tenure and health.

An increasing number of African organizations were promoting social needs of the poor. The Nutrition Society of Nigeria, for instance, reported that "even the most basic staple foods seem to be beyond the reach of the average Nigerian, who now gets less than 80 percent of the recommended intake, with women and children getting even less" (King, 1991). But of course acknowledging a problem didn't always solve it.

What is Africa, Anyhow?

Before entertaining ideas about Africa being a single place with an identity of its own, outsiders shall be reminded that Africa was 53 countries settled by more than a 1000 different ethnic groups — 83 of them in Nigeria alone. Each country had its own language, culture and traditions, each adapting to different geographical and environmental settings in its unique way. Countless numbers suffered or died when foreigners arrived from Europe to exploit the region's fabulous riches: gold, diamonds, copper, ivory, oil and more. Many areas lost able-bodied men and women in their prime to be loaded on slave ships to carry them across the Atlantic or Indian Oceans to the lands of their exploiters. In the case of the Americas, the slave trade lasted more than 300 years, and an estimated 10 million Africans were enslaved. Most of the historic and traditional boundaries between countries, empires and ethnic groups were revised and divided among European imperialists in 1914, with new boundaries satisfying the conveniences of the foreign occupiers. Against such a background, the concept of participatory national governance did not take root.

One well-known historian wrote that conditions for the peoples of Africa were "less favorable to progress than before the colonial invasion had begun: for they had lost their independence and, with it, their capacity to develop along their own lines. They had lost, in short, the command of their own history. At a time when colonial rule was hastening the dismantlement of

Africa's traditional structures, Africans became powerless to begin the building of new structures." And, "even the small minority of Africans who were at last able to achieve a modern education, thanks largely to Christian missionaries, found themselves with a merely peripheral influence on the colonial societies in which they lived" (Basil Davidson, 1987).

Another historian observed that post-colonial Africa had adopted a model of development based on the notion of a centralized nation-state, with Western style and largely Western-owned economic development projects. Consequently, national and regional capitols grew, if not flourished, at the expense of rural Africans and villages. He wrote, "the ambitious schemes by the modernizing elites involved allocating large quantities of scarce resources to urban areas. Rural neglect remained and was even enhanced. Unrelieved peasant poverty was the price for the heavy concentration on the modern sector, on a greatly expanded civil service, and a larger and better equipped army with standards of pay and privileges for the top ranks mimicking those of the expatriate officer class" (Legum, 1999).

Economic Toll

The entire population of highly endemic communities was constantly threatened by malaria. Even those low-grade infections that caused negligible illness still imposed a grievous burden on the victim's immune system. The productivity and prosperity of an entire community were compromised in ways impossible to tally. A reader might remember the mill-man in the U.S. South who wrote to Henry Rose Carter. He told the doctor that his production was 50 percent of normal while malaria occupied the community, and back to normal when the disease was controlled.

One might infer that productivity in Africa could also double if malaria were controlled. Why not? WHO had some startling figures that might be appropriate:

Estimated toll of malaria on African economy (1980-95):

Country	Aggregate loss in billions
Nigeria	$17.3
Congo, Dem. Rep.	$7.1
Ghana	$5.4
Kenya	$5.3
Cameroon	$4.2
Zimbabwe	$4.2
South Africa	$4.1

Source: *World Health Organization* (Lueck, 2000).

Area-specific Strains

Malaria in Africa, as in other parts of the world, was aggravated by movements of people who spread a variety of disease strains across the land. People who had acquired some immunity to the disease from their home areas were virtually defenseless against the new strains. Although war played a major role in the spread of malaria strains, many other opportunities for mixing of populations kept the disease active and dangerous in Africa. For example:

- Agriculturists frequently took pressure off their land by moving to a new area to farm for several years at a time. The practice, known as "shifting agriculture," allowed African farmers to preserve the viability of their crops.
- Some pastoral people moved their animals back and forth between dry season and wet season locations. Often groups met at oases on their routes to allow for socialization and for resting their animals.
- Laborers at Africa's mines also spread malaria infections as they shifted between their homes and their work locations. One of the biggest ongoing labor rotations was at the incredibly rich gold mines in South Africa.

- Religious observances also gave malaria a chance to wreak havoc among some of the most venerable members of the community. In eastern Sudan, malaria was intense in areas where Muslims from many parts of Africa set up camps on their way to and back from the annual Hajj or holy pilgrimage to Mecca, just across the Red Sea.

Epidemiology

In the early 1950s, pioneering work in Africa defined the margins of epidemiology, traditionally known as the study of incidence, distribution and control of disease in a population.

The task was completed by the British scientist, R. Mansell Prothero, whose epidemiological studies defined statistical aspects of human mobility and movement. Among his writings, Prothero produced a popular and illuminating summary of the role of human mobility and movement in the success or failure of disease control.

Prothero had observed several severe outbreaks of malaria in development projects in northwest Nigeria in the early 1950s. As one of the project planners, Prothero described the disruption caused by malaria at new settlements. He said there was clear evidence that the planners gave "insufficient attention" to health concerns. He also pointed out that the wisdom of the period was compromised by an ill-founded certainty that malaria soon would be eradicated (Prothero, 1977).

But malaria outbreaks in parts of Africa that suffered from endemic disease weren't dependent on large movements of people. Just a few children coming home from boarding school a few miles away could bring with them new strains of malaria that might unleash an epidemic.

Oduola's Machine

Meanwhile, back in the university laboratories in Ibadan, one

224

of the senior doctors, Ayo Oduola, demonstrated what were then new diagnostic devices. One new tool was created to assess in advance which drugs may be effective against particular strains of malaria parasites that may be in a patient's blood and which drugs were useless because the parasites had already developed resistance to them.

A sample of infected blood was tested against a variety of available medicines. Within 48 hours, if a potentially effective drug were identified by the test, doctors would be able to start an effective treatment. The doctors hoped the device would reduce the high mortality rates among people suffering from "multi-resistant" falciparum malaria. Such patients wouldn't have to endure the long, dangerous process of trial and error treatments to find a drug or combination of drugs that might be effective.

According to Oduola, an African woman might suffer 10 spontaneous abortions for every two full-term live births. He had compelling personal knowledge about the very high rate of wasted fetuses and the threat to pregnant women among people in his own community in Ibadan. He said, "That's why I specialized in malaria."

Burden of Childbirth

Pregnant women in Africa were at high risk for severe anemia and other health complications, sometimes fatal, in the mother or in the unborn. Remember that the immune system of a pregnant woman was suppressed during pregnancy. Young girls who became pregnant were perhaps at the greatest risk of malaria infections and other complications.

The most dangerous of the complications included maternal and infant anemia, premature deliveries, stillbirths and low birth-weights. Michal Fried and Patrick Duffy, malariologists conducting studies in western Kenya, summed it up: "Malaria acts in concert with maternal anemia to influence fetal outcomes."

Those complications resulted from at least two obstacles to normal blood flow. First was the *falciparum* parasite's tendency to sequester itself in the deep vascular beds of the placenta. In addition, "knobs" or clumps of parasite-infected red blood cells jeopardized the flow of blood to various vulnerable organs.

It was believed that the placenta acquired immunity to *falciparum* parasite over time. Consequently with each pregnancy the mother and the fetus were less likely to suffer from those threats (Fried & Duffy, 1998). Her first pregnancy was the most dangerous to the mother and her fetus. Nevertheless, Fried and Duffy speculated that their research might lead to new treatment strategies. The fact that her immune system apparently offered relief over time from threatening complications suggested to the authors "an attractive target for new therapies." For instance, relief from the adhesion factor associated with *P. falciparum* infections could offer hope to sufferers from cerebral malaria *(Ibid.)*.

Spontaneous abortions or miscarriages were another common complication from maternal malaria. The high, sweltering fever that malaria ignited in a pregnant woman could kill the fetus she carried. Or the fetus could suffer from oxygen deficiency resulting from the presence of parasites-infected blood cells clogging the mother's veins leading to the placenta.

Soon health teams were examining socio-economic factors that hindered effective delivery of health services. Some examples came from F. E. Okonofua and his team who studied maternal malaria among young, unmarried mothers-to-be. They found that while "most people in the community preferred modern treatment of malaria to traditional or religious methods of treatment," that highly sensitive sub-group of unwed mothers tended to stay away from Western-style clinics because of the stigma associated with out-of-wedlock births. Other concerns that jeopardized the delivery of modern care for unwed mothers were the perceived high cost of treatment at the health centers and the lack of privacy (Okonofua, et al., 1992).

Childhood Malaria Takes Toll

At the turn of the century, the greatest worldwide toll from malaria mortality and morbidity were borne by children under five in highly endemic regions in Africa. In fact, by 1999 one of every four childhood deaths in Africa were attributed to malaria (Borst, 1999).[1]

It was known that most people in endemic areas who survived childhood had at least partial protection from malaria symptoms as long as they did not move away from their home community and as long as outsiders with different strains of the disease in their blood did not move in next door.

But many children died before they had a chance to acquire any immunity. Very young children were at highest risk for the disease because they didn't have enough exposure to bestow immunity. They were the ones at risk of severe malaria and death.

One of two common syndromes associated with severe malaria in African children was respiratory distress[2]. That was caused by lactic acid build-up, which itself was caused by severe anemia. Another was the neurological disturbance caused by cerebral malaria. Those life-threatening complications in children could develop very rapidly. The average reported time from the first nonthreatening symptoms to the time of severe symptoms was between 24 and 48 hours. Once in the hospital, many children died despite treatment, and 80 percent of those deaths occurred within 24 hours of admission (Marsh, et al., 1996).

The rising toll of malaria among African children was attributed to the spreading resistance of the *P. falciparum* parasite to chloroquine. Previously, chloroquine was the most affordable and popular antimalarial drug in Africa. But times changed fast. Chloroquine resistance was imposing catastrophic effects on children, according to a 12-year study presented in 1999 at a conference in Durban, South Africa (Pons, 1999).[3]

That research was the first of its kind to quantify the consequence of malaria's evolution in Africa since the first recorded appearance of chloroquine resistance in Kenya in 1979. The study revealed that mortality from malaria in children under five had at least tripled across the continent during a period of 12 years. The statistical study was conducted by Senegal-based researchers of the French institute, Orstom, in three villages in Senegal, West Africa. The findings were corroborated by comparable data from other African countries.

In the Senegalese village of Mlomp, where health campaigns had rendered the use of chloroquine commonplace, malaria killed 11 times more children under five in 1995 than in 1993. But in the remote village of Bandafassi, where chloroquine's use had been limited, childhood deaths only doubled over the same period.

Chloroquine's Power

P. falciparum's drug resistance, apparently starting with resistance to chloroquine, ignited an urgent problem throughout Africa and elsewhere. Kevin Marsh, one of the researchers at Durban, said, "Nowadays you have resistance all over the continent. We need to find urgent solutions." Another specialist said drug resistance in *P. falciparum* was the single most important issue challenging malariologists in Africa at the turn of the millennium (White, et al., 1999).

Nigeria's Ayo Oduola said, "The worst thing is that chloroquine is cheap, useful and available." It was not easy to find a malaria medicine to take its place.

Doctors in several African countries had already switched from chloroquine to the antimalarial drug pyrimethamine-sulphadoxine (PSD). Both cost less than U.S. $0.20 per adult treatment course. But other drugs prescribed for chloroquine-resistant malaria cost more than 10 times that much, beyond the reach of the vast majority of Africans.

Two other factors threatened the lives of children in Africa. Some doctors had been giving contaminated blood transfusions to small children who were dangerously anemic from malaria. The stored blood was at times contaminated with the HIV/AIDS virus and sickle cell.[4]

Dr. Ransome-Kuti

I was able to discuss Africa's urgent malaria status in 1995 with Dr. Olikoye Ransome-Kuti. We spoke in his office at the World Bank in Washington, D.C., where the doctor, a former minister of health for Nigeria, was serving as chairman of the Bank's committee of African health professionals seeking ways to facilitate new programs and policies.

He and I had first met several years previously when I was visiting several African countries seeking guidance for my health education radio programs to address needs of audiences in the developing world who seldom, if ever, got to see a doctor. Ransome-Kuti, a pediatrician, was particularly critical of health campaigns designed and implemented by foreign donors. He believed that the overriding healthcare issue in Africa was "the absence of health infrastructure" — an issue that did not draw much attention among donor countries.

He said, "Although there are many, many tools for reducing mortality and morbidity, the way these tools are delivered to the people is so bad that they never get the full benefit." He specified tools for immunization, water and sanitation, health education, treatment of common diseases and family planning.

Ransome-Kuti suggested several reasons for the shortcomings in public health care delivery. He said, "War and civil unrest often made the centralization and supervision of a national health care system impracticable or in other cases impossible." He said that in some countries, "the unrest is so serious that you just can't work there. And it has set back those countries considerably over the years. All of what they had in terms of a health system has been completely destroyed, and you have to rebuild it."

Ransome-Kuti said corruption also jeopardized the delivery of health care throughout the continent. He said even in times or areas of relative peace, systematic corruption and bribery permeate many African governments from the top echelons right down to the individual health care worker. He said, "If you give the elites a little knowledge, that's what they do; they exploit the poor people."

The limits of basic child and adult education programs in many parts of rural Africa stymied health care efforts according to Ransome-Kuti. That was particularly true, he said, in terms of basic education for African women.

Ransome-Kuti said, "For every datum that we have, it was clear that the mother's education was very, very important for the child's survival. When we analyze the childbirth mortality rate we always find it is the women with the least education who had the highest mortality rate. And it is the women with the least education who used family planning the least. All the data are there."

Western donors woefully under-funded research in disease control and prevention models in Africa, said the doctor. "Thus many health care initiatives were conducted on a campaign basis only."

"It has been very difficult for countries to refuse any kind of offers that people bring to them." He said, "We have complained for years that the kind of assistance they have given us is either what is not needed, or what is needed is done on a campaign basis, not to develop an infrastructure. For example, one donor country wanted to give us money to manufacture sachets for oral rehydration. I said what we need is to teach our mothers to be self-reliant. There is a lot mothers can do to rehydrate their babies without relying on foreign products."

Rural Health Infrastructure

Ransome-Kuti said he came to realize that his goal should be to help rural African villages become self-reliant in terms of basic health care. "Let them see what they can do at a village level. They can't do everything. They won't be able to treat cancer or heart attacks in a village. But they can learn to sort out what they can do and can't do, and refer what they can't do to somewhere else."

He believed a community could develop its own health care protocol at the local level. It should include:

- A health service in every village;
- A referral system run by a community health center;
- Written protocols for personal care, such as washing hands, etc.;
- A structure for a supervisory system to see that everything was managed effectively.

Ransome-Kuti said each new local health aide in an emerging infrastructure would know what she could and what she could not do. The smallest village should have a health aide who merely weighed babies, took their temperatures, and conducted a few other very basic procedures. The aides would refer patients to larger villages when necessary. The system provided conditions that would require the patient to access a more specialized facility when, for instance, a complicated delivery was expected.

A pregnant woman's health care record could indicate how many problem deliveries she had had; how many normal deliveries; her weight and height; and her education level. In some regions, Ransome-Kuti and his colleagues at the level of the regional and national capitols recorded all of the outcomes of deliveries, looking for patterns that might indicate whether a given mother would have a difficult delivery. It didn't sound like much. But simple record keeping could offer valuable protection for the baby and mother.

Sometimes there was a breakdown in management. An example was the immunization campaigns conducted by UNICEF. Ransome-Kuti said, "In my country, 1990 was the deadline UNICEF set to provide coverage to 90 percent of children under the age of two, which we did. But after that, money stopped. Coverage fell. If you had a health system in which you introduced this process, it carries on after the campaign stops."

Keep Pumping

Ransome-Kuti didn't think malaria was Africa's biggest health problem. He said, "Speaking truly, if we really are serious about malaria in our countries we could reduce deaths from malaria by 70 percent, because we know most all of the facts regarding transmission."

Health education for mothers was what was missing. He said that would include, "teaching mothers the significance of fever and the danger it poses to the children and how to treat it immediately. Another step would be teaching about the dangers of mosquitoes to their children and ways to take steps to make sure you are not bitten by mosquitoes. If you really begin to teach our mothers these things they will make sure the children won't die."

"The government can contribute by trying to control the mosquitoes. Various people in the community can contribute by trying to destroy mosquitoes' breeding grounds. But I think the ultimate responsibility will have to be the community, the mothers with the fathers and the village chiefs holding village meetings, going out to inspect their villages."

The doctor continued, "If rural Africans were convinced that mosquitoes breeding close to their homes were the source of their children's illness, then they could take concrete action to correct the problem. Not many villagers know these things," the doctor said. "But they can be taught."

At the time of our interview, chloroquine was still used as a malaria prophylactic and treatment for children. But Dr. Ransome-Kuti opposed reliance on the drug.

"My pediatric colleagues," he said, "were in open arms against me for that. They said, 'Children are mostly at risk between the age of nine months and two-and-a-half years. That's when they die the most from malaria. Now why do you want to put a child at risk of death during that period.'"

But Ransome-Kuti reasoned that "this was the period when children get immunity. If we give them antimalarials, we are just pushing back that period." A baby, in other words, who did not have a chance to develop natural immunity, was critically vulnerable.

"The minute the mother stops her practice of giving antimalarials to her baby, the child will be in danger of dying at every attack of fever. But a baby whose immune system has begun to mature has a good chance of surviving each attack, all the time gaining more reliable control over the disease."

Ransome-Kuti said, "In endemic areas, most people are at least a little sick from malaria most of the time. Rainy season, dry season — the process is there all the time. After five years of age most of us have malaria all the time." He continued, "For example, I haven't taken antimalarials now for more than 20 years. But to maintain my immunity I have to be bitten all the time."

The doctor said, "We pediatricians who treat children are always thinking of this because we know that before reaching five years, the child is at greatest risk for malaria infection." By the time children are in school they may still get fever from a new infection, but they will recover. Adults may never get fever anymore. "You just have the parasites in your blood all the time. If you pump your immune system all the time you can live there," he said. "But if you let your immunity lapse, you're very vulnerable."

Control Projects in Modern Times

For many years, malaria in Africa was considered beyond control. WHO's big dream of eradicating the disease with DDT didn't come close to reaching its goal. What a letdown!

Malariologists found reasons for postponing projects in Africa: The justifiably terrible reputation of the *An. gambiae*, the weak health, educational and economic infrastructures common to many parts of the continent; the abject poverty found in rural areas where the suffering was most intense; and the shifting populations and seasonal migrations that allowed African strains of the disease to spread and thrive.

Gradually, WHO sponsored small pilot programs to try out strategies for analyzing African malaria and to seek ways to ease the burden. Those early separate investigations revealed that a wide range of human factors contributed to the maintenance of high levels of malaria infection. Also, the disease seemed to behave differently at each location — quite an obstacle for experts trying to develop uniform strategies for disease control and prevention!

Traditional grantors were showing reluctance to fund disease-prevention programs that did not offer good odds for success. The reasons were not difficult to understand. Some researchers didn't want to risk their reputations on programs where they could not guarantee good results within a reasonable period. One modern historian was sensitive, even eloquent, on that topic. He wrote, "It would be hard to fault [...] the early battlers against malaria for putting to one side the major problem in order to define a smaller one, one they could hope to deal with. A crusade for human life, organized selectively, could easily become a defense of the privileged [...]. The technical difficulties of helping the black masses could easily serve to excuse complacent neglect. And sometimes did. Yet it is hard to see how the first fighters could otherwise have retained the optimism to act at all and so to keep alive the possibility of extending the fight later on."

Protection With a New Face

As early as the 1930s, some malariologists had been recommending that young children in Africa should not be treated for their first attack of malaria. For instance, malariologist S. P. James suggested in 1932 that malaria control strategies should allow the patient to acquire immunity against the disease (James, et al., 1932), even to the point of allowing the well child to be deliberately exposed to the disease.[5]

As Ransome-Kuti recommended later, it would be in the interest of the child and of the community at large to allow him or her to suffer from malaria early in life. If the child were not sufficiently infected at an early age, he might not develop immunity during the small window of opportunity provided by the mother's antibodies.

WHO was encouraged, however, by what at first seemed like success with residual sprayings with DDT. The agency did not acknowledge the gravity faced by young children. The agency did begin more than 20 pilot projects throughout Africa during the mid 1950s and early 1960s. But none of the new pilot projects yielded the quantified epidemiological data that was crucial to planning malaria control strategies.

Garki Project

Meanwhile, some members of the scientific community were losing confidence in the expectation of total mosquito eradication with DDT. Malaria epidemics were appearing in tropical regions, mostly in Asia, that had been sprayed with DDT. In 1969, WHO decided to abandon its expectations. The agency chose instead to look for alternative strategies. Three techniques for controlling malaria were examined — indoor household spraying of DDT, massive in-home drug administration and collecting and analyzing data on the quantitative dynamics of malaria transmission; that is, assessing the information being gathered.

The exploratory data were examined in the Garki district in northern Nigeria, a location selected because it had among the highest documented prevalence and incidence of new malaria infections anywhere. The region under study consisted of 164 villages located 100 kilometers northeast of the city of Kano. The two largest participating ethnic groups were the agricultural Hausa and the pastoral Fulani.

The studies, done from 1969 to 1976, recorded and monitored malaria figures before and after interventions with antimalarial drugs and indoor spraying. The findings confirmed poor results of earlier studies in the Sudan savanna, northern Cameroon and in the Upper Volta (now Burkina Faso) area. While the application of residual insecticides — in that case, DDT — did indeed kill lots of mosquitoes, it did not bring about any reduction in malaria.

Roll Back Malaria

The poor results at Garki, as well as the disappointments of the Alma-Ata initiatives, failed to provide hope for malaria reduction in Africa. Nevertheless, by 1998, WHO specialists were ready to launch a new worldwide program that seemed to involve the same familiar strategies and hubris of the earlier massive malaria control projects. The new project was called Roll Back Malaria or RBM for short. It promised to cut in half the worldwide malaria burden by the year 2010. As announced, the new campaign was "an opportunity not only to beat a devastating disease, but also to develop endemic countries' health systems and build new means of tackling global health concerns" (WHO, 1998).

The new worldwide campaign focused first on Africa, with comprehensive goals:
- Upgrading health delivery systems at local and national levels in malarious countries;
- Developing new drugs for victims already infected with malaria;
- Coordinating the development and testing of new malaria drugs and vaccines;
- Intensifying the use of impregnated bed nets to prevent nighttime biting by infected mosquitoes (*Ibid.*).

At the time, it was known that most victims of malaria died simply because they did not have access to health care close to their home or because their ailment was not identified immediately as malaria. In addition, lifesaving drugs often were not available. In Africa, RBM planned to create a network of teams to go into villages to analyze treatment and prevention practices at the household and community levels.

Another goal of Roll Back Malaria was to set up a resource network throughout Africa to forecast malaria epidemics and plan for their prevention. The network would link surveillance information from countries and regions to coordinate projects. Also, under the umbrella of Roll Back Malaria, an independent foundation was established for the sustained pursuit of the discovery and development of affordable antimalarial chemotherapies into the 21st century. That endeavor was called "Medicines for Malaria Venture" or MMV for short. It was based on a partnership among several public sector agencies, philanthropic organizations and the pharmaceutical industry. In 1999, three major drug discovery projects involving academic and industrial groups were selected for funding at a combined total of $4 million per year through MMV.

Bed Nets

As part of its Roll Back Malaria campaign, WHO announced in October 1999 a drive to provide nearly 60 million African families with bed nets treated with a "relatively gentle" insecticide, pyrithrum. The bed nets would be distributed over a period of five years.

Bed nets had been used for disease control by several ancient civilizations, including Egypt, Rome and India (Najera, undated pamphlet). The application of residual insecticide to fabrics as a means of personal protection against vector-borne diseases just began during the Second World War with the impregnation of bed nets and combat clothing by the Soviet, German and U.S. armies.

In the 1970s pyrethroids were used for that purpose; their high insecticide activity, combined with their allegedly low mammalian toxicity, made them ideal for treating fabrics, according to project sponsors.

A scientific panel convened in 1983 by WHO had reviewed the first laboratory evidence, and it recommended field trials to assess the potential of technology for disease control (Lengeler and Snow, 1996). One concern was that the nets would develop small rents and tears allowing insects to penetrate the fabric. Periodic rinsing with insecticide seemed to correct the problem.

Studies in a number of sub-Saharan countries that used insecticide-treated bed nets revealed that child mortality rates in some regions were cut back. In fact, a study of five regions of Gambia with a total population of 116,000 indicated use of insecticide-impregnated bed nets might reduce by 25 percent the mortality in children aged 1 to 9 (Brown, 1999; Mann, 1999).

But other studies painted a more solemn picture.

Bed Nets Critics

An article in the journal Science stated that insecticide-treated bed nets were shown to prevent only one death in every 200 children who used them (0.5 percent) — an efficacy rate significantly lower than those from the studies used by WHO to support their bed net program (Ochert, 1999).

A computer model created the same year at Oxford University offered another view. Epidemiologist Chris Newbold and his colleagues reported that children could acquire lifetime immunity against malaria if they are bitten once or twice during their first year by infected mosquitoes (*Ibid.*). That seemed to confirm what Ransome-Kuti and others had been saying all along. They had maintained that effective clinical immunity would develop only after a given amount of exposure to malaria. The authors warned that decreasing exposure to mosquitoes would prolong that time and "would increase susceptibility to the severest forms of falciparum malaria" (*Ibid.*).

It was also believed that under certain circumstances a control campaign with bed nets could do more harm than good. In the late 1990s, a study was released questioning the long-term effects of control measures that were based on reducing malaria transmission in endemic areas. The controversial rationale was discussed by malariologists for more than half a century, but the timing and scope of the new proposal and the professional stature of the authors drew new attention to the issues.[6]

The authors explored the connection between severe malaria morbidity and the level of parasite transmission in 3,556 children. The study covered three to five years in five communities in Gambia and Kenya. Findings supported the seemingly paradoxical observation that the risk of severe malaria in children was lowest in places where the disease was most active, and was highest in places where malaria displayed low to moderate presence. Also, in communities with highest malaria activity, the risk of severe disease was greatest only during the first two years of life, whereas in communities with lower malaria activity, that period lasted until age five (Snow, et al., 1997).

Another issue raised by some researchers was the accuracy of statistics. Numbers don't lie. Nor do they tell the whole story. In regions lacking basic health care infrastructure, accurate reporting of health status presented a major challenge, as the reader was aware. Tabulating figures of people sick with malaria could be quite accurate because the blood tests were reliable. But determinations of the causes of death were not reliable.

Young children in most parts of Africa were threatened by a number of life-threatening diseases such as infant diarrhea, tuberculosis, measles, upper respiratory tract infections and AIDS. But what actually killed the victims was a puzzle.

Another issue in many malaria control campaigns, as in other campaign-based health programs, was that local people would be receiving general health and nutrition education. Any drop in mortality or morbidity may be due to the general increased awareness of people about their health. Changes in health practices like diet or cleanliness could be recorded as part of the drop in mortality due to the use of pyrithrum-treated bed nets.

Finally, there was one issue that always concerned someone like myself — the nervous mother of four children. I would have been reluctant to let my children sleep under bed nets dipped in insecticide.

Where Is the Truth?

I am reminded often of Mark F. Boyd's remarks in 1941 addressing the Symposium on Human Malaria sponsored by the American Association For the Advancement of Science in Philadelphia: "Unfortunately, students of modern medicine are but slightly, if at all, conversant with the older writers, particularly those preceding Laveran, and thus fail to appreciate the substantial character of the contributions which have come down to us from the past" (Boyd, 1941).

Perhaps we can hold it all in balance, the new and the old. Remember, the new will be old before long. And maybe malaria will outlive it all.

---

[1] Some investigators indicated that, a more accurate figure of malaria deaths might be closer to one out of every two children (50 percent of childhood deaths) in many areas (Marsh, et al., 1996).

[2] Defined as difficulty in breathing. Clinical manifestations included cyanosis (a bluish tinge under nails and skin due to lack of oxygen), severe retraction of chest wall with every breath, an increased respiratory rate, and an expiratory grunt.

[3] The four-day conference was held under the auspices of Multilateral Initiative on Malaria (MIM), a program aimed at developing medical exchanges between the Northern Hemisphere and Africa.

[4] See pg. 123 for more on sickle cell.

[5] The same view was expressed by N. H. Swellengrebel in later years.

[6] The study was co-authored by thirteen scientists and appeared in June 7, 1997 issue of *Lancet*.

Chapter 10
Southeast Asia

W AR ALWAYS PROVIDED lessons in geography. For instance, how many people in the U.S. knew before the 1960s where Vietnam was? Now it's practically part of our heritage.

My own family was living in New Delhi, India, when my husband Charley's office in New York assigned him to go to Vietnam and report on the new simmering war. I had to turn to the atlas to find Vietnam. I imagined Americans everywhere reaching for the atlas. Soon we all knew that Vietnam was in Southeast Asia, or, as it was commonly known before World War II, Indochina or French Indochina. I learned later that the region was home to virulent malaria and that geography and environment were critical in defining the disease.

For the purposes of examining malaria in Southeast Asia, I decided to focus on Vietnam, Cambodia, Thailand, Myanmar (formerly Burma), all on the mainland and finally Sri Lanka (formerly Ceylon), the island nation near India. That would allow me to take advantage of some enlightening reports from a regional WHO meeting in New Delhi in 1991.[1]

Mountain Barriers

The mainland of Southeast Asia was scored by thickly forested north-south mountain ranges descending from Tibet to the flatlands and wide deltas along the South China Sea, allowing isolation and safety for separate countries or kingdoms dating as far back as 2000 years. Each closed-in population had developed independently with unique customs and histories. Each country had its own ethnic orientation, religion, currency, language, systems of authority, governance and customs for succession.

Foreign traders were attracted to Southeast Asia since the early 16th century. The attractions included the convenient, safe and strategic waterways between China and India, the unexploited natural resources, the masses of cheap labor and potential for sustaining large plantations for foreign markets. One big attraction was the spice trade. Eventually, the region was colonized by five world powers that seldom functioned outside the centers of power. But, as foreign traders as well as missionaries streamed in, local cultural differences remained intact.

Myths and Reality

Each country also had its own creation myth or myths. One creation myth of Vietnam seemed to hold a thread of truth. The myth related the marriage in 2800 BC of Vietnamese Prince Lac Long Quan to a fairy named Au Co. She gave birth to 100 eggs and each hatched, giving the parents a total of 100 sons. Then the parents separated. The mother took her half of the brood across the northern mountains, while the other half followed their father into the Red River Delta. Historians have pointed out that the story very well could symbolize the two early branches of the Vietnamese people (SarDesai, 1994).

Vietnam extended for L,200 miles along the Tongking Gulf almost as long as the entire Pacific coast of the continental U.S.. It was like two heavy baskets on either end of a carrying pole. The "baskets" represented Tongking, which occupied the Red River Basin in the north, and Annam, which held the Mekong river basin in the south. The two were separated in the middle by the coastal dynasty of Champa.

Tongking apparently was settled first. In ancient times, it was occupied by so-called Negrito-type people anthropologically resembling tribes of Indonesia and Polynesia. They were followed by Mongoloids who migrated south from the lower Yangtze valley in China and usurped prime territory, pushing the earlier arrivals into the mountains where many made their homes in caves. Each of the three regions was developed separately by aggressive dynasties driven by territorial needs and competitive nepotism.

China's Grip

Early Tongking with its enviable rice culture soon grew too prosperous for its own good. China seized the province as its own and held it for more than 1000 years, from 111 BC until 939 AD, an accommodation described by historians as a "love-hate" relationship. Both sides benefited. China acquired a wide buffer against attack from the south and more room for its expanding dynasties.

The relationship with China offered benefits to Vietnam as well. Vietnamese people were able to learn Chinese healing skills, Confucian social and political values, Mandarin bureaucracy and civil service examination system, and the arts of language and literature. And, perhaps most importantly, the Vietnamese people were able to absorb agricultural technology and flood control strategies for application in the Tongking Delta. Vietnam had already created an elaborate system of dikes and canals. China contributed its own techniques of dam construction and the maintenance of a compartmentalized field system to protect rice fields from flooding (SarDesai, 1994).

Those irrigation techniques were still practiced widely and profitably in the 150 square miles of flooded plains near Haiphong in the Red River Delta when I was there in the mid-1990s. Perhaps the only difference between the rice fields of historic times and the modern day bucolic scene was the presence among the rice of new family shrines honoring war dead. But shrines to war dead were ubiquitous to the region through history.

Another early benefit China provided the Vietnamese people was protection from outsiders. One historian said: "The more they (the Vietnamese) absorbed of the skills, customs, and ideas of the Chinese, the smaller grew the likelihood of their ever becoming part of the Chinese people. In fact, it was during the centuries of intensive efforts to convert them into Chinese that the Vietnamese came into their own as a separate people with political and cultural aspects of their own" (Buttinger, 1968).[2]

Mongol Invasions

Throughout history, evidence abounded that Vietnam was able to defend itself against enemies. Take, for instance, its defense against multiple invasions of the infamous nomadic Mongols. Beginning with Genghis Khan in the early 12th century, generations of Mongol conquerors came out of Mongolia and swept across most of Asia, creating one of the most expansive empires in history.

The Mongols established the Yuan Dynasty (1279–1368) in China, conquering most of the neighboring areas including Burma and Korea. But their three attempts to conquer Vietnam between 1257 and 1285 were unsuccessful (SarDesai, 1994).

One of the earliest stories describing the importance of what was probably malaria in Vietnam involved the last of the Mongolian invasion attempts. To secure trade routes to India and

Persia, Kublai Khan sent his son Togan in 1285 to conquer the Red River Valley. After several months of failures, the Mongols gave up, defeated by the "climate" — a word often used for malaria (Ognibene and Barrett, 1982, citing Kiel, 1968).

Malaria had always been a serious problem in Southeast Asia, especially in the forest highlands. In Annam, the southernmost section of the country, the disease apparently had been known for thousands of years and was ascribed to evil spirits in the mountains. People said the spirits lived near the water and attacked men during sleep. Persons with malaria were described by the popular phrase *mat bung, da chi* or "pallor of the face with slatelike tint" (*Ibid.*).

Peace With China

The two adversaries, China and Vietnam, learned the art of coexistence, which worked most of the time. The rare uprisings were short, except for the period between 1407 and 1428 when the Ming armies of China overran Vietnam, dragging it back under direct Chinese rule. Anyone familiar with the inimical history shared by the two parties would have expected fireworks. But the two sides apparently had acquired a kind of self-serving tolerance. One historian described it as a "subtle interplay of resistance and dependence, which appeared often to stand at the root of historical Vietnamese attitudes toward the Chinese" (SarDesai, 1994, citing David Marr, 1971).

Missionaries in Action

The presence of French people in Vietnam starting in the early 17th century invited new political complications. The French were not successful traders, unlike the Dutch. Historians pointed out that the French court frequently complicated trade policy. But missionaries from France were very successful, especially the missionaries at Fai Fo mission south of Danang.

At the beginning of the 18th century, missionaries claimed more than a quarter million converts to Catholicism in coastal Vietnam. One French missionary, Alexandre de Rhodes, created a method of writing the Vietnamese language in Roman script, making communications easier for most outsiders.

Another French priest, Pigneau De Behaine, assumed an activist role in Vietnamese politics. The internal political climate of the period was stormy and highly nepotistic. The Nguyen family controlled all of Vietnam, with its power base in Hue in central Vietnam. Three brothers ruled separate regions, but one died without naming an adult heir. Fears arose that the Nguyen power base might be seized by a rival dynasty, the Trinh family from Tongking. That seemed to threaten the safety of the leading heir to the Nguyen family, Nguyen Anh, who was whisked to Annam for safekeeping.

His young son, Nguyen Canh, joined De Behaine on a trip to France to seek help from the court of the "Sun King," Louis XVI. It would be hard to choose a less propitious time. France was facing its own political turmoil. The fall of the Bastille was a month away. Nevertheless, Louis directed the colonial governor in Pondicherry, India, to provide needed assistance.

The troops, however, were not provided, and De Behaine raised the money himself for 300 troops and for several shipments of arms. By the time the new troops arrived, Nguyen Anh was already strengthening the fortunes of the Nguyens. He captured Saigon (now Ho Chi Minh City) in 1788. He secured the important Hue in 1801 and took Hanoi a year later, ending four decades of conflict between the Nguyens and the Trinhs.

Once the kingdom was secured, Nguyen Anh reorganized it into three divisions and 26 provinces linking the entire coastal route between Hanoi, Hue and Saigon, a distance of 1,300 miles that could be covered on horseback in 18 days. That earned him recognition as the unifier of Vietnam. With those victories behind him, Nguyen Anh proclaimed himself emperor of Annam with the title of Gia Long (SarDesai, 1994).

Malaria Scorecard

European troops stationed in Vietnam during the 19th century learned to respect the destructive power of Southeast Asian malaria. The French army physician Alphonse Laveran[3] reported that between 1890 and 1896, 25 percent of the European troops stationed in Vietnam died of malaria. During the period 1945 to 1954, a total of 293,814 cases were recorded, although only 620 deaths occurred. The incidence of the disease, however, showed a progressive decline during that period. In 1946, the incidence was 40 per 1,000 troops per year; it had dropped to 9 per 1,000 per year by 1954 (Ognibene and Barrett, 1982, citing Kiel, 1968).

France Extends Its Reach

France soon intensified its commitment to dominate Southeast Asia. One prize would be a chance to dominate the entry to China by way of the Tongking Gulf (SarDesai, 1994). In 1881, the new French Premier Jules Ferry justified the conquest of Tongking saying, "It is not a question of tomorrow but of the future of fifty or a hundred years; of that which will be the inheritance of our children, the bread of our workers. It is not a question of conquering China, but it is necessary to be at the portal of this region to undertake the pacific conquest of it" (*Ibid.*).[4]

A series of skirmishes that followed ended with the Treaty of Tientsin of June 9, 1885, recognizing the French protectorate over Annam and Tongking. France was granted preference over all European powers in Yunnan, the Chinese province across much of the northern border with Tongking. Also, France was given the right to construct a railway paralleling the Red River Valley from Hanoi to Kunming, China. As historians have pointed out, the treaty marked the extinction of the nearly two-millennia-old subordinate relationship of Vietnam to China (*Ibid.*).

Two Wars

War and global politics in the 20th century left their marks on Vietnam:

1945:
- At the end of World War II, the victorious powers helped evict the Japanese forces that had occupied Vietnam. In fact, the Allies utilized the Japanese forces to keep order until the French could get back.
- Ho Chi Minh proclaimed independence from France for all dissenting Vietnamese.
- French forces arrived to take back Vietnam by force, drawing on support from various leaders from southern Vietnam, the U.S. and from several European powers.

1946-54:
- The Vietminh[5] and the French fought a bitter nine-year war known as the First Indochina War.

1954:
- The Vietminh defeated France at the Battle of Dienbienphu, and the French gave up their colony for good.
- The U.S. assumed France's role with a pledge to halt the spread of communism in Asia.

1975:
- The Vietminh forces defeated the U.S., ending the 30-year struggle for independence.

Writer's Block

It was difficult for an American writer to touch only briefly on the Vietnamese-American war. I must assume the reader has access to libraries and bookstores or the Internet, offering a small mountain of accounts of the traumatic, controversial period of our history. Our book remains restricted to the role of malaria in peace and war, with enough background to illuminate the environmental and social setting that sometimes seemed to connive with the disease.

"Jungle Tax"

After the U.S. assumed France's failed attempt to regain control of its colony, the Vietminh realized they needed a reliable transportation and communication link with the South. An old network of highland trails or paths used mostly by tribal people covered the entire western length of the colony, running roughly parallel to the Truong Son mountain range. In 1959, the Vietnamese began an ambitious plan to upgrade the trail to provide safe movement of Vietminh troops and heavy equipment. By then, U.S. strategists were setting up a string of intelligence units in South Vietnam. There were 28 posts in all, roughly shadowing the old trail, which lay, to the west.

To the Vietnamese, the route soon became known as the 'Truong Son Road,' or 'Duong Mon Ho Chi Minh'; in the West, however, it became famous — or infamous — as the 'Ho Chi Minh Trail' — so named by the French Army (Tang, 1985). By any name, the trail was an engineering feat that eventually was credited with the final victory over helicopters, B-52 bombers and the best war machinery money could buy. In addition, the trail was a thoroughfare for malaria, allowing drug-resistant strains of the disease to proliferate and play a role in wartime strategy.

The trail stretched from Hanoi to Saigon, snaking in and out of neighboring Laos. At first it took trekkers as long as six months to travel the distance from the north to the south. A "transportation group" of about 50,000 Vietnamese workers was responsible for modernization and upkeep of the trail. First, they hard-packed the trail with clay or crushed rock. Loads of 250 to 300 pounds were slung on bamboo poles on both sides of bicycles pushed by porters. According to some accounts, the record load weighed 900 pounds (Shaplen, 1986).

To build up their strength before starting a trip, trekkers were given double or triple the standard ration for several weeks. On the day of departure, each person was loaded with a pack weighing between 70 and 80 pounds, and each carried in addition a rifle or carbine. Packs included extra clothing, a hammock, a plastic sheet for rain protection, and often a part of a heavy weapon. A tube of rice — called an 'elephant intestine' — hung around their necks (Chanoff and Toai, 1986).

Even all that preparation did not prove adequate to appease the environmental hazards of such a septic jungle in the early stages of the trail's construction and maintenance. Those included leeches, poisonous snakes, dysentery, malnutrition, jaundice, pneumonia, the plague and malaria (Lanning and Cragg, 1992).

None was as great a hazard as malaria. Incidents of malaria were so frequent and severe that some troops came to refer to the disease stoically as the "jungle tax." One soldier, for example, wrote in later years, "for each of my years in the jungle, I spent approximately two months in the hospital, battling the high fevers and general debility of the disease." Almost all the jungle dwellers were marked by a rather recognizable jaundiced and sickly appearance. In fact, on more than one infiltration mission, their sick demeanor gave the guerrillas away (Tang, 1985).

It was estimated that up to half of the deaths that occurred in the region during the early years of the war were related to malaria. In 1971, Dr. Pham Ngoc Thach, North Vietnam's minister of health, visited the trail to conduct research on malaria prevention and control. He died on the trail from malaria that same year (*Ibid.*).

A number of factors were responsible for the severity of the disease along the Ho Chi Minh Trail, factors common through history to areas all over the world. The forested mountain slopes the Trail passed through already had the highest malaria levels in the country. In fact, malaria of the highland forests of Southeast Asia apparently was about as bad as a disease can get.

As one would expect, the mosquito population was continuously disrupted by the modifications to its environment: removal of trees and shrubs to widen the trail or to create new spurs, or placement of new surfaces, and, later in the war, the addition of bomb craters. Thousands of new pools of water were created, attracting displaced mosquito populations. Mosquitoes, of course, could adapt to disruptions by altering their lifestyle. The result was new generations of more versatile and sturdy mosquitoes for transporting the malaria parasite. Troops were given antimalaria medicine with their meals throughout the journey. But the medicine apparently wasn't any more successful among Vietnamese people than it was in people from the U.S..

During the late stages of its wartime history, the trail had changed from a scattering of dirt paths to a highly developed network of over 10,000 miles of trail. It included over 600 miles of double-lane surface that accommodated trucks and other heavy military vehicles. Movements of materiel had risen to levels surpassing 10,000 tons of supplies per week. And a trek that would have taken six months in 1965 took no more than 10 days by 1974.

Better maintenance of the roads and the decreased time any one given soldier would spend on the trail were critical factors in the drop in the incidence of malaria. Deaths on the trail attributed to malaria dropped from 50 percent to 15 percent by the end of the war. That, of course, was still a heavy toll. By contrast, despite the most massive bombing campaign in world history, only one percent of combat deaths on the trail were bombing-related, making the cost to the U.S. for killing one soldier by bombing an estimated $1 million (Unpublished research by writer John Pursell, 2000).

Research Units Deployed

While the communist government in the North was upgrading the Ho Chi Minh Trail for heavy wartime use, U.S. military physicians were upgrading their defenses against malaria. Doctors experienced with the disease had been convinced by the terrible losses to malaria in World War II that they needed to be better prepared for any future military mission in Southeast Asia.

But by the time the formal surrender for that war was signed on the battleship Missouri in Tokyo Bay on September 2, 1945, high-level strategists in Washington believed the biggest future threat to U.S. security would not be in Asia. Major emphasis in military planning was focused instead on Western Europe for several reasons. Political instability in Europe was obvious and ominous. The post-war partition of Germany and Berlin, and the controversial Soviet acquisition of several Eastern European countries led U.S. planners to expect their forces and medical support units to be serving in Europe in the near future (Dirks, 1972).

The U.S. did, however, establish a medical unit in 1946 in Japan to serve the needs of U.S. occupation forces. The unit was strengthened when North Korea launched raids into the south in 1949 and 1950, and was strengthened further when the raids escalated into war. The Korean War (1950–1953) brought American troops once more into contact with malaria, precipitating a surge of drug experimentation.

Several successful — or at least temporarily successful — drugs were created, including new drugs for treatment of malaria or for prophylaxis. The new malaria drugs were effective, however, only for vivax malaria, which was common in Korea. That species of the parasite was a lot easier to subdue than the potentially deadly falciparum malaria farther south.

The scope of U.S. military medical services continued to widen to accommodate virtually all laboratory disciplines in the Far East command, including laboratory support in the field, epidemiology and entomology, with an emphasis on disease vectors.

A U.S. Army medical research team was invited to join a project on scrub typhus at the research facility of the Malayan Medical Services of the British Colonial Government in Kuala Lumpur.

Later that facility came under U.S. direction and was renamed the U.S. Army Institute for Medical Research (IMR), in Malaysia. The institute expanded its work with malaria and mosquitoes.

Alarm and Complacency

Meanwhile, the success in Korea against vivax malaria was contributing to a comfortable complacency among some international medical professionals about the outlook for malaria in general. In 1961, the WHO reported that "the clinician had at his disposal a complete series of effective drugs for the treatment of all stages of the disease." Malaria research was continued, nevertheless, in the hands of prescient military medical personnel with close familiarity with falciparum malaria and with the foreboding encroachment of drug-resistant strains.

Colonel Tigertt

Colonel William Tigertt was one of those prescient U.S. Army physicians with a strong influence in guiding policy forward, developing new drugs and mastering the idiosyncrasies of *P. falciparum*. He had seen malaria in the Philippines and New Guinea during World War II and was aware of emerging reports of drug-resistant *P. falciparum*. He also had a deep knowledge and respect for history and a taste for literary eloquence that appeared in his own writings. An example was a quote from poet-philosopher George Santayana (1863–1952): "Progress, far from consisting in change, depends on a retentiveness... When experience is not retained, as among savages, infancy is perpetual" (Tigertt, 1966). He was referring of course to the misguided periodic celebration of victory over malaria.

Tigertt made his first visit to Vietnam in 1961 while he was on temporary duty at IMR in Kuala Lumpur. Coincidentally, that was the year of the WHO claim that doctors had all the malaria medication they needed and also the year the first resistant strain in Thailand was identified. In Vietnam, he was leading an exploratory team analyzing future needs if the war were

253

to escalate. Tigertt created strategies for protecting troops from the kind of misery U.S. forces had to endure in previous wars where armies were not adequately prepared for malaria.

Two years later Tigertt was appointed director of WRAIR in Washington, D.C. Malaria in Vietnam was on track to become the Army's biggest medical problem. Most of the cases were traced to the forested highlands along the Ho Chi Minh Trail. In addition, the disease was spreading fast.

Army Doctors Respond

Tigertt and his team of Army physicians and researchers responded to the malaria alarm in several ways. Their goal was to discover why so many troops were coming down with the disease in spite of the fact that each service person was issued chloroquine and primaquine weekly.[6] The two drugs in one pill had always been effective in the past.

Tigertt authorized new treatment or convalescent facilities throughout South Vietnam so troops with malaria didn't have to be evacuated to the U.S. or to new hospitals in the Philippines or Tokyo for skilled treatment. He introduced new diagnostic and treatment protocols, upgraded the skills of technicians to process thick blood smears needed for diagnosing malaria quickly, and he contracted civilian labs in the U.S. and elsewhere to identify where the new strains might be coming from.

One of the most important links in analyzing the foreign strains was Dr. Robin D. Powell of the University of Chicago Army Medical Research Project at Stateville Penitentiary in Joliet, Illinois. Powell received blood slides from Korea and Vietnam to identify specific strains of *P. falciparum* that might be responsible for the growing number of individuals who did not respond to the standard treatment. Powell and his associates also were able to test new and old medicines against blood specimens from a variety of locations in Vietnam. They recruited volunteers from the Illinois penitentiary to submit to injections of parasites to learn more about specific strains of the disease and to seek a cure.

During the mobilization for the defense against malaria, scientists screened an estimated 300,000 compounds (Tigertt, 1990). None was both effective and safe. The magnitude and obstacles of the WRAIR drug search reminded Tigertt of a parallel. Before the U.S. entered World War II, President Franklin Delano Roosevelt ordered an urgent program for building warships to help Great Britain keep its sea-lanes open. Roosevelt said if the U.S. could build ships faster than the Germans could sink them, the Allies would win the war. Tigertt could relate to that. He said his goal was to create medicines faster than the parasites could acquire resistance.

But warships, as history would demonstrate, were easier to build than an effective, safe malaria medicine.

New Drug Fails

One drug introduced for malaria prophylaxis and treatment was dapsone, a sulfa compound used successfully since 1949 for treatment of leprosy. Doctors at leper colonies in parts of Africa had observed that lepers taking dapsone had a lower incidence of malaria than did other individuals in the community. In the early 1960s, investigators in India and Nigeria had found that a single dose of dapsone produced a clinical cure in semi-immune patients with malaria. After a U.S. Army research team confirmed the positive results, dapsone was combined with other drugs and tested in closely monitored field trials in Vietnam. Researchers were optimistic that they at last had discovered a drug that would control battlefield malaria.

At first, all was well. Individuals on dapsone suffered fewer cases of malaria or milder symptoms or shorter episodes of symptoms. But problems surfaced. In one group, 16 soldiers who took dapsone developed agranulocytosis, a critical shortage of certain white blood cells. Eight of them died from the reaction and use of the drug was halted or altered (Ognibene and Conte, 1982; Hembree, 1980).

Irregulars and Special Forces

The forested highlands and plateaus of Vietnam were home for several communities of tribal people known collectively as the Montagnards, a French word meaning mountain people. The Montagnards stayed in the forests and made their living mainly from forest products. They were alienated from the main stream of Vietnam, but tourists might see postcards in hotel lobbies featuring the exotically dressed people who didn't look at all as if they belonged in Vietnam.

The Montagnards were a crucial source of help to U.S. intelligence units providing clandestine surveillance along the shadow of the Ho Chi Minh Trail. The qualifications of the Montagnards were impressive. They were unobtrusive, almost to the point of blending with their environment. They had already worked for the French surveillance missions and knew the region intimately. And since malaria was endemic in their home territories, it was assumed the Montagnards were immune from the disease and didn't have to take weekly prophylaxis. But that was not a safe assumption. In fact, that was a dangerous assumption — dangerous for the Montagnards and dangerous for the U.S. Special Forces they worked for.

The U.S. Special Forces, or Green Berets, were a U.S. Army unit established during World War II to assist Yugoslav resistance forces. It was not unlike spying. The Montagnards conducted a variety of assignments for the Special Forces. They were attached to one or another of the 28 Special Forces camps monitoring movements of Vietminh or other bases set up in remote western areas. Typical duties included reporting troop movements and changes in the enemy's behavior. They also were organized to collaborate with and train local people as agents and to assist other Special Forces units that were facing difficulties.

Typically, the Montagnards spent several weeks at a time patrolling an assigned region. Then they returned to base camp to be "debriefed." In military language, their units were called CIDG companies, or Civilian Irregular Defense Group. They were the "irregulars." Sometimes they were called "Ms" for Montagnards, or "MIKE" forces.

The routine suffered breakdowns early in the war. The scouts were susceptible to sudden attacks of acute malaria, as if their lifetime immunity to the disease was switched off. The pattern was consistent. The agents would leave for a surveillance mission of several weeks. But after just several days in the field they often experienced the familiar symptoms: chills, shaking, fever and pain. Tests by the base camp's medical unit confirmed the suspected diagnosis: falciparum malaria. It was an aggressive, potent strain or strains, and recovery was slow.

The victim apparently was bitten by an infected mosquito soon after he left base camp. After an incubation period of five to seven days the disease struck. There was no compromising with the infection. The victim was incapacitated until the disease ran its course.

It was obvious that the *P. falciparum* causing all the trouble was new to the region. The human carriers were among the enemy units entering the region for the first time. The strains of malaria they brought with them were new to that area. The local people had no experience with those strains, like new babies with their first exposure. Once infected, the victims could become carriers themselves. And they did. Both groups, the "irregulars" and the Special Forces, suffered acutely and were unable to carry out their assignments.

The chain reaction of infections that followed did not provide any new lessons for treatment or prevention strategies. But some patterns started to appear. The ground fighting near the Cambodian border was the most heated, and the numbers of casualties seemed to reflect the destructive tide of engagements.

Fort Bragg

One early encounter with aggressive malaria from the high-lands of Vietnam took place in an Army hospital in the U.S., the Womack Army Hospital at Fort Bragg, North Carolina.

Col. Llewellyn Legters, a physician with the Green Berets, was stationed at Bragg in 1964 after he returned from temporary duty in Vietnam. His assignment in Vietnam had been inspection of Special Forces bases in the highlands with his colleague, Col. Craig Llewellyn.

Later, during his stint at Bragg, Legters had under his care a serviceman home from Vietnam. He remembered that the patient had the familiar symptoms — fever, pain and chills. The patient had completed his tour of duty at a base near the Cambodian border, not far from Saigon. He apparently became infected with malaria before leaving Vietnam, but the symptoms did not appear until he was home.

Blood slides confirmed he had falciparum malaria, and Legters treated him with chloroquine. When that didn't help the patient, Legters telephoned Dr. Powell in Chicago for advice. Powell recommended treatment with quinine, which helped but only temporarily. The disease kept recurring.

Powell also asked Legters to send him a blood specimen from the patient. The specimen was administered experimentally to a volunteer at the Illinois penitentiary for further testing. The results were sobering. The patient was harboring a rare and particularly virulent strain of *P. falciparum.* That was one of the first clinically proven cases of drug-resistant malaria.

Several years later when I talked to Legters in Washington, D.C., he told me the failure to get a response from the medication "scared the hell out of people" at the hospital. "Here was a parasite that was not only resistant to the antimalarial drugs that we were using as prophylaxis but relatively resistant to quinine," he said.

The patient eventually recovered.

Legters' Plan

Craig Llewellyn returned to Saigon where he was a surgeon for the 5th Special Forces group, and Legters was preparing to present their new proposal asking for a cross-disciplinary team of infectious disease specialists, epidemiologists, technicians and others.

Their goal was to discover the origin of the unusual *P. falciparum* strains and to understand how to protect the troops. Legters said, "Lots of things were going on without trained observation."

Legters' next challenge was to present the proposal to Tigertt, who held the purse strings for WRAIR during that period. Tigertt had some characteristics familiar to his subordinates. A meeting could be especially unsettling to an officer with a proposal to present, said Legters. He remembered, "All the time that you're nervously making a presentation to get his approval of a big new project, he's sitting with his back to you, feet propped up. There is a silence while you're standing there not knowing what he thinks of your idea. Then he swings his chair around and simply asks 'How many spaces?' I told him we needed 26 on our team. And I got 26."

Legters and his new 26-person staff would be attached to the U.S. Army Special Forces — Walter Reed Army Institute of Research. They were called the Field Epidemiological Survey Team (Airborne) or "FEST" for short, and they assembled in Vietnam in the fall of 1966. The team moved up and down the length of South Vietnam obtaining blood smears from Montagnards suffering from severe clinical malaria.

Their first mission, which Legters called "ill-starred," was a search for North Vietnamese army incursions along the Cambodian border.

Team members in Legters' group examined the Montagnards before they left the base. About 30 percent of them had parasites in their blood, but were judged "perfectly well." After they reached areas near North Vietnamese army units however, the Montagnards began to suffer. Upon their return to the garrison they developed clinical attacks of malaria.

"This told us MIKE force were susceptible to clinical attacks in spite of the fact that they were supposed to be semi-immune," said Legters. And it told them as well that there was considerable morbidity amongst the forces as a consequence of malaria; that the strains were being imported from outside, by way of the North Vietnamese Army; and that they might benefit from prophylaxis. "The assumption had always been that there was no benefit to be gained from prophylaxis because these people were semi-immune. And so they were protected, as opposed to U.S. troops who needed prophylaxis," said Legters.

Legters added, "What this showed us was that strain differences in falciparum malaria from place to place and from population to population were what was causing clinical attacks of malaria among indigenous troops." He said, "Their semi-immunity was not protecting them from the reservoir of North Vietnamese Army. The strains that were being imported were resistant to chloroquine, and we needed to have prophylaxis for indigenous troops."

I asked if the captured troops from North Vietnam were free from malaria.

He said emphatically, "No. They were sick. There was no question about that. I don't think I have ever seen sicker people in my life functioning. They were shivering with chills. They were a sorry bunch when they were taken prisoner… suffering from the same strains as the U.S. forces. They acquired their malaria coming down the Ho Chi Minh Trail. And the malaria drugs they had at their disposal weren't protecting them either. Not any more than chloroquine by itself was protecting our troops…"

"What medicine did they have?"

"They had everything under the sun. In other words, whatever they captured, whatever they could get from whatever source. And they had a hodgepodge — chloroquine, palludrine... a host of antimalarial drugs. Whatever they had in stock at the time a unit departed with from North Vietnam, from any direction — that was the drug that was issued. I think their malaria problem was contracted on their way down from North Vietnam, west of Vietnam in Laos."

Counting the Patients

The tally of U.S. Army casualties attributed to malaria at the 8th field hospital in Nhatrang, reflected the trends:

Number of malaria casualties treated by year:

1963–1964	39
1965	1,972
1966	6,662
1967	9,124
1968	8,617
1969	7,322
1970	6,718

Seventy-two malaria deaths were recorded, from 1965 to 1970, averaging out to about 13 deaths per year (Barrett, 1982).

Ia Drang Valley

The U.S. sent 200,000 troops to Vietnam in 1965. And by spring of the following year, American troops were ready to launch their first big offensive against enemy forces in a dense jungle of the Ia Drang Valley near Pleiku. The operation was called "Silver Bayonet" and was designed to stop infiltration into South Vietnam by troops from the North. It was perhaps the most intense ground fighting until that time. The U.S. troops were supported by helicopters and B-52 bombers. The casualties were very high.

The U.S. lost more than 300 troops. The North Vietnamese reportedly lost almost 2,000.

The battle was viewed by the U.S. commanding officer as a victory, but viewed by many Americans as too high a price to pay for the strategic advantages claimed (Karnow, 1983; Barrett, 1982). Public opposition to the war was growing.

Collecting Mosquitoes

According to Legters, vector species and behavior were difficult to analyze. "It was a bit of a logistics problem because the field collection of mosquitoes were done at night, usually inside a perimeter of defense of some sort. We had to conduct man-biting collections, meaning that someone sits with his pants legs rolled up or sleeves rolled up with some portion of his skin exposed. And then someone sits there with him and as he reports the presence of a mosquito, a red filtered flashlight would be flashed on — red to avoid the attention that a light would attract in the jungle. Then the aspirator simply sucks the mosquito into a vial."

I asked, "Did you ever offer yourself up for the duty?"

"Oh, sure. Hell, we were being bitten all the time anyway. This was just a little more systematic way to get at how many mosquitoes bit during an hour. What time of day do they bite? What time of the evening do they do it?"

"Did you ever get malaria?

"No. In fact none of my team did, except one, because we were on preferred prophylaxis. Once the mosquito was collected, then it went back to a laboratory where it was dissected and the infection rate was based on finding sporozoites in mosquitoes that were dissected. That was the logistics of it. You do the man-biting collections at night in the jungle or in a perimeter of defense, and those mosquitoes in vials in boxes would be loaded on the first helicopter, a re-supply helicopter coming in the morning, back to a more definitive laboratory where the dissections were done."

"Your team kept moving from one location to another?"

"There were people in the field, people operating out of a camp west of Pleiku. There were people in Pleiku. The whole system was designed to supply this operation. After several weeks in Pleiku for the initial study, we would start follow-up studies to work on some of the things we had learned."

Tet Offensive

Beginning in early October 1967, malaria among Montagnards and U.S. forces was intensifying, indicating a build-up of troops from the North. The outbreaks were spreading south along the border with Cambodia and terminating around what was called the Seven Mountains Area. Previously, falciparum malaria was sensitive to chloroquine. But in the last few months of 1967, the Americans had been aware of a heavy increase of drug-resistant strains of the disease.

Legters said, "It made us think there were North Vietnam army troops nearby." There were indeed a lot of North Vietnamese troops nearby, about 70,000 of them, all along the Ho Chi Minh Trail. They came prepared to inflict simultaneously so much damage in so many areas that the U.S. would seek an end to the war.

That was the "Tet Offensive" of January 31, 1968. "Tet" was the Vietnamese Lunar New Year, celebrated by feasting, gift giving and family reunions. The sudden orchestrated attacks were made against more than 100 cities, 13 of the 16 provincial capitols in the Mekong Delta, and the Saigon area. The city of Hue, with its ancient citadel, received the most intense assault and was held by the Northern forces for 25 days. The other targets were penetrated but held only briefly by the attackers. At the time, some observers believed the attack totally destroyed the U.S. ability to win the war. In retrospect, historians in modern times were saying the same thing (Karnow, 1983).

Malaria Closes the Camp

Malaria casualties were gradually diminishing. One investigator, however, reported details of a battle in 1969 that he called "a classical example of a sizeable military force being rendered combat-ineffective by malaria." Major Stephen C. Hembree was in Long Hai, southeast of Saigon, in 1969 at a camp established mainly for the defense of a military airport. The location, a coastal plain, was not like the typical stricken areas in the highland forests. But there was one similarity. Both locations attracted considerable malaria.

The site was one of the 28 Special Forces camps, and it also was the site of a CIDG company of Montagnards. The company suffered a 59.7 percent rate of asymptomatic malaria. That meant that 59.7 percent of the men harbored parasites without suffering the symptoms of the disease. They could function as required. After the mission, 31.7 percent of them were very sick with malaria and could not perform their duties. The immunity acquired from a lifetime exposure to the parasite was not effective. It was reminiscent of the experiences of folks everywhere who lost their immunity when they were exposed to certain foreign strains of the disease.

Hembree's survey included several posts over a period of two years. A malaria outbreak in Long Hai resulting from exposure of troops in Long Khan Forest southeast of Saigon was "one of the most extensive and explosive outbreaks known to have occurred among the CIDG," wrote Hembree.

The total force was about 2,000 men, and their forward operating base was an abandoned airstrip. After one engagement, the battalion commander said in his report that the operation had been halted because of the toll due to malaria.

Post-war Health Care

The number of U.S. casualties due to malaria continued to drop as the end of the war drew near. Several reasons were offered for the decline. U.S. doctors were learning more about what to expect when a patient displayed indications of chloroquine resistance. Also, American forces were initiating fewer ground missions, the kind of missions that exposed troops to malaria carriers. The new U.S. strategy was to attempt to wear the enemy down with air attacks.

According to some international health experts, the care provided by the communist forces in the North was functioning well. After the war, medical relief missions from various donor countries and nongovernmental organizations helped Vietnamese professionals establish or modernize various treatments and care facilities. Vietnamese scientists also collaborated on projects in other countries to explore new treatments and drugs against malaria.

More Testing for Artemisinin

Trials in Vietnam provided evidence suggesting the potential role of artemisinin derivatives in the control of severe malaria and its associated mortality. A sharp decline in malaria mortality levels was observed in the country following the introduction of the artemisinin derivatives. At the time, however, no pharmaceutical company was willing to pursue development and full registration of those drugs. Return on the investment was just too low.

WHO launched a new initiative in public health delivery in 1999 with the development of artesunate, which was believed to be the most efficacious of the artemisinin derivatives. An artesunate Task Force was set up to operate as a "virtual" pharmaceutical company, meeting twice a year to oversee the development of artesunate with the aim of providing national programs with additional means to control malaria. Its members included the University of Cape Town in South Africa, WHO and other experts and regulatory officials.

Community trials were organized in several countries to

evaluate the efficacy of rectal artesunate in emergency situations. It was believed that early administration of artesunate rectally might halt severe disease and prevent a fatal outcome. That information was required before the FDA approved a wide-scale drug trial. In addition, the trials were expected to provide a platform for subsequent development of health education programs in the new millennium.

Health Care in China

The Chinese Communists won their own civil war in 1949. That was followed by their early public health projects with preventive and curative campaigns that drew the attention of various international public health specialists. In fact, many of the most basic aspects of the Alma-Ata health initiatives were drawn from the Chinese experience. The chief of the World Bank's Education Policy Division, Dean Jamison, summarized China's early emphasis on the basics.[7]

The government devoted 3.3 percent of its annual budget for 1981 to financing health care programs. According to Jamison, "While great variation in financing arrangements exists throughout the country, in general, the State and communal levels combined with self-help finance the greater part of the preventive measures, leading to relative uniformity of their distribution around the country" (Jamison, 1987).

First came a project for the elimination of four common pests that spread disease — rats, flies, mosquitoes and bedbugs. In a mobilization starting in 1951 under the aegis of China's National Patriotic Health Campaign Committee, successful malaria control projects had been launched. Jamison said, "The reduction in the incidence of malaria has been largely due to campaigns to fill in stagnant ponds and eliminate other mosquito breeding sites."

Other points mentioned included China's creative financing for health infrastructure. Jamison said that China's health care planning relied on lower-level staff, committees and individuals — as opposed to highly trained and expensive professional health care providers. In addition, attention was given to improving the country's water supply, sanitation, public health education programs and nutritional levels.

Gifts From the Forest

Some scientists believed that groups of pre-human primates, their parasites and mosquito vectors evolved in highland forests in Southeast Asia.

It was believed also that thalassemia and other red blood cell disorders that apparently evolved as protection from malaria appeared in Southeast Asia.

In more recent times, the isolated tribal people who lived in the core forest areas of Southeast Asia were very poor and never benefited from the advantages of the development around them. But they typically had some acquired immunity to the strains of malaria in their restricted environment.

In many ways, however, life on the forest periphery was more hazardous than life in the core of the forest. On the periphery, the "constant ebb and flow of a large floating population," engaged in wood gathering, gem mining, forest agriculture and ethnic/political migrations, promoted proliferation of mosquitoes and the diseases they carried (Sharma & Kondrashin, 1991).

Vector's Advantages

The high level of adaptation acquired by mosquitoes allowed them to continually evolve into strains better capable of dealing with new pressures humankind placed on their environment. Two general modes of protection were recognized in mosquitoes: chemical and behavioral. They could produce specialized enzymes to neutralize chemically the threatening substances, such as insecticides in their environment. Or, they could modify their feeding schedule or other habits to avoid the environmental dangers. It was clear that the emerging strains of mosquitoes in Southeast Asia were benefiting from both kinds of protection. Experts reported that "no real progress in malaria control could be achieved in spite of continuous spraying of insecticides for many decades" (Sharma & Kondrashin, 1991).

In addition to the mosquito, the parasite itself had rapidly evolved to deal with threats in its environment. At the turn of the millennium, decades of large-scale sub-optimal use of antimalarial drugs in Southeast Asia had continuously selected for hardier parasites that were resistant to virtually all the commonly used antimalarials (Ballou, 1994).

Cambodia

To the west of Vietnam was Cambodia, a hot bed of malaria. Most of the population traced their ethnicity back to the Khmers who built a powerful empire in Southeast Asia around the ninth century, an empire that lasted for many centuries. The Khmers were influenced by the culture of India and erected numerous monuments that remained standing into the 21st century.

Cambodia had tremendous resources, a region of mines and rubber plantations, with migrant workers carrying various strains of the disease. It also was a haven for North Vietnamese troops at the end of the trek south on the Ho Chi Minh Trail — a safe place to assemble and prepare for sorties across the border into Vietnam. The troops brought in strains of malaria from all along the trek.

In 1975, as the North Vietnamese forces were on the eve of their victory over the U.S., Cambodia erupted with one of the most violent civil wars in modern history. The Khmer Rouge[8] guerillas took over the country, and waged a war against urban intellectuals who eventually were forced into the countryside. Thousands walked west to bordering Thailand and stayed in refugee camps, while others were able to enter the U.S. and other countries offering asylum. An estimated 1.7 million people, or more than one-fifth of the country's population, died or were killed while the Khmer Rouge were in power.

It would be a challenge to imagine a setting more conducive to the proliferation of malaria — civil war, multiple migrations, mining, forestry and poverty. Malaria was rampant with new strains developing rapidly.

But Cambodia had already been recognized for years for its notorious malaria. The gem-mining town of Pailin in Cambodia near the border with Thailand, was one of the first areas in the world where drug-resistant *P. falciparum* strains were detected. As early as 1957, subsequent to mass distributions of medicated salt (chloroquine added to table salt), chloroquine resistant *P. falciparum* were identified in the area.[9]

In 1973, it was reported that some workers in the Pailin area were no longer healed by the available combination drug therapies for malaria. By 1981, resistance to the commonly used sufadoxine-pyrimethamine combination therapy had become widespread in the area.

When mefloquine was developed, researchers tried to limit its use to lessen the risk of emerging resistance. But mefloquine apparently remained unchallenged in Cambodia for only six or seven years. On his 1992 visit to the affected areas in Cambodia, Jean-Paul Menu, WHO's special health envoy, remarked that although mines were perhaps killing two to four people a day, malaria was killing very many more" (Rensberger, 1992). The rapid appearance of drug resistance there continued and the Cambodia-Thai border became one of the first locations of multi-resistant falciparum malaria. The parasite had become adapted to all the antimalarial drugs on the market.

Based on the geographical and chronological progression of drug resistance in Southeast Asia, some scientists hypothesized that the Cambodia-Thai border was the "epicenter" for drug-resistant falciparum malaria in Asia. However, there was also evidence to support the theory of an inherent and independent development of resistance in different geographic locations.[10]

Thailand

Thai means free, and the Thai people took their freedom seriously. Historians traced the origin of the Thai people back to their homeland in the Yunnan area of southern China. The area of modern day Thailand was part of the Khmer Empire in the 13th century, when the Thais began their major migrations southward. The Thais took control of the area with the Thai state gradually establishing a prominent position in the region (SarDesai, 1994).

Thailand was among the most prosperous of Asian countries. It was one of the world's leading producers of rice, besides having coal, gold, lead, tin, rubber and precious stones. Thailand was unique in Southeast Asia for escaping domination by outside powers. It was never colonized. But like other countries of the region, it was not able to control the malaria in its highland forests.

New strains of *P. falciparum* apparently were introduced into Thailand by the almost continual migrations of mineworkers and refugees from the Pailin area of Cambodia and from Thailand's western border with Myanmar. As in Cambodia, by 1981, resistance to sulfadoxine-pyremethamine treatment was common in Thailand. But the Malaria Program of Thailand was very active in conducting studies and introducing effective new combination drug therapies.

Due to its political stability, Thailand was for many years, the final destination of waves of refugees from neighboring countries. The government maintained many refugee camps in various border locations. For example, the Shoklo refugee camp near the border with Myanmar was one of the locations chosen for trials of the Pattaroyo vaccine.[11]

Myanmar

Myanmar, an agricultural country with great natural resources, was known as Burma until 1989 after a military government took over. The same factors that contributed to high levels of malaria in other countries of the region have been present in Myanmar.

Forests there covered more than 40 percent of the land. DDT residual spraying was used against mosquitoes for 30 years without success. Typical of their behavior elsewhere, mosquitoes developed resistance to insecticides in Myanmar. Most of the malaria cases reported were from the forest or forest fringe areas, and the remainder primarily from population diffusion and migration along international boundaries. As in other poor tropical countries, development projects like dam construction, road construction and oil exploration, disrupted the natural balance of mosquitoes' environment in the forests, and also gave malaria parasites an opportunity to spread their strains over an expanding population.

Falciparum was the most common malaria infection in the forests and its proportion declined in the plains or urban areas, but the parasite had become resistant to chloroquine.

Sri Lanka

Sri Lanka, the island nation south of India, was known through history as the land of gems. It was said that King Solomon procured a great ruby for the Queen of Sheba from Sri Lanka. Another famous gem from Sri Lanka was a 400-carat blue sapphire, misnamed the "Star of India," which was on permanent display in the Museum of Natural History in New York City.

Sri Lanka was also known for its pattern of virulent malaria for centuries (Wickramasinghe, et al., 1991). For much of that time the disease erupted every five years.

People relied on various strategies for killing mosquito larvae until residual spraying with DDT was introduced in 1946. A quick drop in malaria was reported but the disease returned, in some places worse than before. Spraying campaigns were renewed in 1959. By 1962, DDT sponsors believed Sri Lanka seemed to be on the brink of total victory against the disease. But the toll of the disease began to rise in 1965, slowly at first but steadily. Then in 1968 and 1969, figures soared. Half a million people were reported stricken. After more spraying in 1972, cases decreased to 150,000, only to increase again in 1975 to 400,000. As forested areas were cleared for development, mosquito populations and malaria victims soared again. By 1991, about three-fifths of the population were malarious *(Ibid.)*.

Failures of the spraying projects led to a growing lack of public acceptance for spraying in Sri Lanka. Other unfavorable factors were high cost, possible health hazards and the realization of the evasiveness of mosquitoes. Experts in Sri Lanka came to the conclusion that malaria should be controlled in a different manner. Attempts were made to develop an integrated vector control strategy that minimized the use of insecticides.

Recommendations were made for new control strategies that would be flexible and diversified, specifically suited to local conditions. Those new strategies needed to be easily sustainable by the local population and updated frequently based on fluctuating epidemiological assessments. With the rapid environmental changes in the peripheral areas created by socioeconomic developments, there was a rapid change in the mosquitoes' behavior. That meant the relevance of entomological data that was used in the past had to be questioned.

Something New

Malaria in Southeast Asia was a very old phenomenon, particularly in the forests. It was an ecological disease and required a solution based on various ecological parameters throughout Southeast Asia. As the end of the millennium was approaching, it was becoming evident that temporary intervention measures were incapable of interrupting the incredibly well-adapted disease. Such measures could actually do more harm than good. In addition, development projects that cut deeper and deeper into the ancient forests of Southeast Asia promoted new malaria. There was an apparent consensus that development strategies should be planned with consideration to public health problems and that cross-border collaborations were extremely important.

By the late 1990s, WHO had already begun projects based on new understandings. Also, a notable regional collaboration was launched by the Asian Collaborative Network for Malaria (ACTMalaria), an independent international organization with the goal of improving training and communication on malaria. The organization was formed in November 1996, and in 1999 membership consisted of representatives from nine Southeast Asian countries.

Since 1997, ACTMalaria was working with WHO in projects to provide annual fieldwork and training courses known as Management of Malaria Field Operations (MMFO). The objectives were to provide knowledge and experience in malariology and malaria program management.

Some observers pointed out that Asia's problems were being solved by Asians, a long stretch from the days when international health programs were designed by outsiders under the assumption that 'one size fits all.'

---

[1] Sharma, V.P. and Kondrashin, A.V., *Eds*, (1991) *Forest Malaria in Southeast Asia*. Proceedings of an Informal Consultation Meeting WHO/MRC, 18-22 February, 1991, New Delhi.

[2] From *Vietnam: A Political History* by Joseph Buttinger, 1968, Praeger, New York.

[3] Discoverer of the malaria parasite in 1880.

[4] From *Jules Ferry and the Renaissance of French Imperialism* by Thomas F. Powers Jr. as quoted by SarDesai, 1994.

[5] A contraction of the names of the two leading groups seeking national independence: the Vietnamese Independence League and the Indochinese Communist Party.

[6] Chloroquine was the antimalarial used successfully all over the world since 1943. Primaquine was one of the drugs used successfully against vivax malaria in Korea.

[7] Jamison's analysis was presented at a conference on *"Good Health at Low Cost,"* sponsored by the Rockefeller Foundation. It appeared in a Rockefeller Foundation book of the same title.

[8] French for "Red Khmers," so called after the Khmers.

[9] Chloroquine was added to table salt in Cambodia, parts of South America and sub-Saharan Africa. Chloroquine was the only antimalarial used by most national malaria programs and was given by mass distribution to entire populations (Kogstad, 1996).

[10] See 'Drug resistance' on p. 145 for more details.

[11] See 'New vaccine is tested in the field' on pg. 165 for more details about the trials.

Chapter 11
Fire In The Amazon

MALARIA WAS RAGING out of control in the Amazon Basin since the beginning of the 1980s, the largest localized epidemic in modern times. I spent five weeks in 1990 traveling in the region looking at specific problems. I crisscrossed through four of the Amazon states in Brazil,visiting remote communities, field hospitals and clinics, and research institutions.[1] I talked to doctors, nurses, public health workers, entomologists, biologists, sociologists and social workers, engineers, and sick people and their family members.

A conservative guess of the number of people with the disease in the Amazon then was 1 million. Nobody really knew how many people were sick. A commonly used rule of thumb there was to double the number of cases reported, which was about 600,000 in 1990. Authorities assumed that fewer than half of the people who were sick with malaria actually went to the clinic and were counted in the records. The death rate was unknown, but was believed to be lower than it was with other malaria epidemics throughout history.

Observers believed that a great many lives had been saved by the dedication and ingenuity of Brazil's unusual cadre of public health workers.

The new epidemic began in the 1960s when Brazil's federal government encouraged the landless poor in the southern and central states to settle in newly deforested regions of the Amazon. By 1980, the epidemic was spreading like a flash flood, overwhelming the region's thinly distributed public health services. And by the late 1980s, there was no sign of abatement.

Most of the victims were among the several million new settlers who had no natural immunity against the disease, since malaria had been virtually eradicated long before in their former home areas. Large expanses of the Amazonian rain forest were being burned and cleared, and the resulting ecological disruption had triggered a population explosion of mosquitoes. The insects were more than normally aggressive in their quest for human blood because the forest mammals that they had fed on had vanished in the smoke of deforestation. Another major locus of malaria transmission was the miners. According to The New York Times, in 1990, more than half a million small-scale, freelance miners, or "garimpeiros," were digging and panning for gold and cassiterite[2] along the banks and bottoms of many tributaries of the Amazon (Brooke, 1990).

Stone Age Tribe

During that leg of my journey I was traveling with Dr. Leonidas Sales Sampaio, a malaria specialist from the large inland port city of Manaus and with a public health inspector from Boa Vista, the nearest city. Sampaio, who had invited me to join him on this field expedition, was a senior physician for SUCAM, Brazil's public health service for malaria control. Leaving from Manaus, our first stop was Paapiu village, a remote community of Yanomami Indians in the northern reaches of the Rio Mucajai near the border with Venezuela.

The Piper six-seater rocked in the turbulence over the hills near the settlement as the river below sank from view into the green jungle. The plane started its descent, banked to the right and seemed about to land on a cushion of treetops. Finally, the wings leveled, and the trees parted to reveal the landing strip, an irregular, slightly uphill, unpaved path.

Our bouncy landing was watched by a group of Yanomami Indians, part of what has been called Brazil's largest surviving Stone Age tribe. A number of villagers came out to greet us. The small people of Paapiu village didn't look at all like the people in the old TV documentary I had seen the night before in the exit lounge at Manaus International Airport. Those TV Indians had been expressionless, with immaculate, uniformly coifed hair and with painted faces and sharp twigs stuck through their cheeks. Wearing grass aprons or penis shields, bright feathers and traditional jewelry, they had performed somber, shuffle-step-hop dances and mock hunting pantomimes with their long bows and arrows. They didn't look real. The Paapiu villagers on the other hand were real people. While a few of them had paint on their faces and sticks through their cheeks, they all had that casual and disarrayed look of very poor people anywhere who don't have enough to eat, who don't have much choice about what to wear, and who don't have much to do.

The Yanomami were recent victims of the malaria epidemic. Until recently the disease had been practically eradicated in Brazil. But now, malaria was erupting all over the Amazon basin. The Yanomami communities were a textbook example of the way the disease selected its victims. The jungle their ancestors had inhabited since Neolithic times was full of malaria, but the malaria parasites, the mosquitoes and the Indians had existed in a kind of triangular equilibrium. All three were part of an old, evolved harmony. As long as they remained isolated from the outside world, the Indians had been able to tolerate the strains of the parasite common to their region.

Equilibrium turned to chaos in 1987 when the garimpeiros came to the Yanomami region. Apparently the miners, who had been crisscrossing the Amazon for many years, carried in their blood strains of malaria to which the Yanomami had never been exposed. The techniques the garimpeiros used to extract gold and cassiterite from the river's tributaries were responsible for the new standing pools of water where the mosquitoes were breeding. With help from the mosquito vectors, the strains of malaria brought by the miners had mingled with the indigenous strains carried by the Yanomami. Both groups suffered from the new outbreaks of malaria, but the Yanomami were hardest hit. Approximately half of the Indian population was suffering from the disease when I was there. Earlier in the epidemic the proportion was even higher.

Missionary Nurse

On deplaning, we were greeted by the missionary nurse, Sister Irma Guilda Maria Rauber, whose wide and radiant smile seldom left her face. She looked like a tourist, in her T-shirt, shorts and sandals. She had flown here from Porto Alegro in the south of Brazil under the sponsorship of FUNAI, the country's agency for Indian affairs, to help the people of Paapiu survive the worst part of the epidemic. Other Yanomami scowled on the sidelines or scurried back to their shacks on the far side of the "runway." In addition to their own traditional dwellings, they had taken over the makeshift shanties that had been abandoned by the miners, those ubiquitous structures made of cardboard, wooden crates, and bright blue plastic tarpaulins. Sister Irma explained to us that the Indians didn't like visitors because they thought that any outsiders could bring new malaria, as the garimpeiros did. The Indians were convinced the new severe malaria had arrived with the miners who had just left a few days prior to our visit. But the Yanomami found it hard to believe that the female mosquitoes could simultaneously extract blood from and inject malaria into a person's flesh, or that the insect's saliva was the mode of transmission. According to the nurse, they believed instead that outsiders gave them malaria by clicking cameras at them.

A few women and young children clung to Sister Irma and her two assistants as we all walked to the "shabono," the Yanomami word for their traditional large communal houses. The new shabono was a convalescent hospital the Indians had recently built for themselves. The huge circular structure, which was eight meters or so in diameter, was strikingly beautiful. Its high, curving walls were graced by the same blue tarpaulin sheeting that poor people throughout the Amazon and all over the developing world used for their temporary dwellings. The roof of the convalescent shabono was thatched with forest branches and looked from the outside like the "big top" of a small town American circus. Indeed, the roof was high enough for a high-wire act. Graceful ribbons of smoke from the many small fires inside rose through the rafters.

Jungle Hospital

As we entered the shabono we saw that it resembled a military hospital close to a battlefield. It was very quiet, dark and smoky. The little light that penetrated the rafters showed us first the traditional hammocks that hung higher up, some suspended. Then slowly the lower hammocks became visible. The dismal scene that gradually emerged from the smoke and shadows resembled a faded sepia photographic plate from the American Civil War. The shabono's hammocks were filled with tier upon tier of the very ill people. Some of the hammocks were clustered in what seemed like family groups.

Sister Irma explained that 40 or so malaria patients were housed there, along with other family members who cooked for the sick and helped to care for them. Then, as our eyes began to focus more clearly, we saw Yanomami women crouched over small, smoldering fires. Many small fires, one apparently for each family group, were spaced across the dirt floor. Some of them were being used to cook meals for the patients, while other dying fires smoldered unattended.

Perched high on a wall in a strip of daylight, a small monkey watched our every move. We remembered that some monkeys could be infected with their own, nonhuman kind of malaria, strains that apparently did not make them sick. And we remembered reading somewhere that certain Indian communities kept monkeys around their homes as a kind of decoy for the mosquitoes. Those ravenous insects would bite just about any warm-blooded animal at hand. But a FUNAI official later dismissed that theory, "Any monkeys the Yanomami keep around the house are for their dinner," he said.

Sampaio, a gentle, quiet man with a boundless sympathy for all the people of the Amazon, started to examine some of the children who lay wide-eyed and listless in their hammocks. He called me to the side of one 6-year-old boy: "Do you see the size of his spleen? He's obviously very anemic." The spleen, an organ just under the ribs on the left side, acted like a sponge, removing dead cells from the blood. In addition, it helped make special white blood cells that destroyed disease agents such as the malaria parasite. The boy's protruding spleen was swollen to the size of a football. It was hard and unyielding to the touch.

Death Rate Stays Low

Sister Irma then escorted us back down the path past the runway and showed us the two-room hut that served as the Paapiu public health clinic. The front room was the dispensary, its walls holding several shelves of medicine and medical equipment. The second room she called "the infusion room." She explained to the doctor that the incidence of malaria among the Indians in Paapiu had declined from nearly 90 percent during the height

280

of the epidemic to the current level — roughly 5o percent of the population was sick at any given time. Death rates had been high, the nurse said, but nearly everyone recovered quickly.

A fast response to the infection, in terms of both diagnosis and treatment, apparently was crucial to the control of malaria in this village and region. I remembered that the single-cell malaria parasite would multiply thousands of times in the first few days of infection. By the time symptoms had developed — the classic fever, chills and pain — the typical patient had been infected for more than a week, and there would be millions of parasites in his or her red blood corpuscles. Sampaio told me later that "If you treat it at the beginning, nobody dies of malaria." But millions of people around the world, most of them children, had indeed been dying from the disease. Diagnosing malaria at the very onset of its symptoms, and having effective drugs on hand for treatment, was impossible in most parts of the developing world not fortunate enough to have the close attention of a health specialist.

The Indian community at Paapiu was unusual in other ways. It was small enough to allow the missionary nurse to know to the day when each new patient began to show symptoms of malaria. She would do a blood test immediately. As soon as the blood was dry, the nurse could read the slide under her microscope, and she knew exactly what she was looking for. She could easily recognize the distinguishing features of the malaria parasite and recognize as well which species of parasite — *P. vivax* or *P. falciparum* — had caused the infection. Here, as everywhere else, *P. falciparum* was the species that most often caused grave or fatal complications and the species that was quickly acquiring resistance to the medicines traditionally used as a cure.

Close Monitoring

Under ideal circumstances all malaria patients would be isolated quickly, before mosquitoes could suck up infected blood and pass it on to other, healthy people. Such isolation of people with malaria was almost impossible in most endemic regions, but not in Paapiu. Indians sick with malaria stayed in the shabono for at least two weeks while they recovered from their infection. The nurse said that virtually no mosquitoes were able to enter the structure, despite the fact that it didn't have any screens. Practically no field hospitals and clinics in the Amazon could afford the screens. But Sister Irma believed, as did most of her Indian patients, that the pungent smoke within the shabono was an effective mosquito repellant.

Another requirement for successful malaria treatment was surveillance of patients. Sister Irma personally monitored each of her patients to ensure that he or she was indeed taking all the medicine she had prescribed. She administered one drug for patients suffering from vivax malaria, and a different one for *P. falciparum* infections. If recovering malaria patients were not closely supervised, they might not complete a course of medicine. Some drugs tasted bad, and others had unpleasant side effects. Patients were tempted to abandon the treatment as soon as the symptoms had started to abate.

If the patient were comatose or felt too nauseous to swallow the medicine, Sister Irma could administer the medicine intra-venously in the "infusion room" of the clinic.

Malaria and Gold

Sampaio and I sat down with Sister Irma and other members of our entourage in the clearing by a cashew tree to talk about malaria control among the garimpeiros. The missionary nurse didn't know why the miners had left Paapiu only a few days before. But they certainly hadn't gone far; they were working several kilometers downstream at a new "garimpo."

Garimpeiros had been mining gold from the streambeds of Brazil since the 18th century. Typically, a prospector traveled throughout a wide area looking for indications of gold. He did spot checks of stream sediment with his *baiteo*, a conical pan that tapered to a small point in the center. The prospector swirled river sediment around and around until the heavy gold particles sank into the small tip in the bottom. If he did find gold, he would return to his base and bring in more people with some slightly more advanced technology. Historically, the garimpeiros had traveled Brazil's maze of rivers and tributaries by boat. More recently the preferred mode of transport was plane or helicopter.

Once a promising site had been chosen, the miners were ready to operate on a bigger scale. They dug sediment from the banks and bottoms of the river or sucked it up with a powered vacuum machine. The raw material was then mixed with mercury to bind with any gold that was present. When the treated sand was shaken, sieved and washed again, the heavy pieces of gold-mercury alloy were easily identified and removed. Then the mercury was burned off with a gas torch.

The pure gold was weighed and purchased by any one of a number of merchants in a nearby town. In about a year, the garimpeiros would have all the gold they could retrieve with their simple technology. They would then move on, taking their profits and their malaria with them.

Miners Accepted, To a Point

Garimpeiros were usually well-tolerated in the towns. Their total production accounted for an estimated 90 percent of Brazil's gold income, and Brazil was the world's third biggest producer of gold, after the former Soviet Union and South Africa. The garimpeiros were big spenders while their luck held, and local businessmen didn't mind having them in their areas. Most of the time, of course, they were out in remote places where there was nobody to bother.

Sometime within recent years word spread that the hills around Yanomami country were full of gold. An estimated 40,000 garimpeiros came to the region from all over northern Brazil and southern Venezuela, and probably from other places as well. But here their mining activities were not well-received. Only about 20,000 Indians remained in the area, descendants of the far larger migrations from North America an estimated 15,000 years ago. Their culture was still largely Neolithic, and they had little contact with local or federal government or others.

The reaction of the town folks to miners was not at all tolerant when reports started reaching the rest of the country and then the rest of the world that the gold miners of Brazil were invading the reserves and the culture of the Yanomami, destroying their environment, and poisoning their streams with mercury. Killing the Indians with foreign strains of malaria was seen as an additional offense.

Brazilians had become sentimental, almost paternalistic, about the Indians of the Amazon, who were suffering a lot of genocide, venereal diseases, and other contagious diseases from outsiders. Brazil's paper money, the Cruzada, had a picture of a Yanomami on it, and pullover shirts with Yanomami-related themes were available in shops throughout the country. The president of Brazil at that time, Fernando Collor de Mello, was being pressured by other governments and political groups all over the world to take action to protect the Yanomami and their environment.

The pressure dovetailed with growing international criticism of the widescale burning of the Amazon rain forest for settlement and development projects. A number of Brazilians who had settled in this region, many of whom were alienated and isolated from the rest of the country, felt that the president was anxious to demonstrate to foreign environmentalists that he supported them. He had to do something, his critics said, and it was too late for him to undo the damage of the fires. So two months after his March 1990 inauguration, Collor ordered the army to dynamite the miners' airstrips. Many of them were destroyed, and the president promised to keep up this action as long as was necessary.

Gold Production Drops

Some miners simply rebuilt their landing strips. Others returned to their garimpos by helicopter. But many of them did leave. Several months after the raids of the landing-strip, about 20 percent of the original estimated 40,000 miners had left the area. Gold production dropped by almost 70 percent, and the informal marketing that supported the industry started to deteriorate.

Observers claimed that the miners were ready to move anyway and that the president's initiative was merely an added incentive. There may have been several other reasons for leaving. The culture of the garimpeiros was inherently unstable. The miners were plagued by alcoholism, violence, and territorial feuds. Also, miners reportedly were afraid of the Yanomami and didn't like living in such close proximity to an alien people who fought among themselves and were good marksmen with a bow and arrow. It was possible as well that the miners were simply running out of promising or viable sites. Perhaps they had heard about a big new unexploited area elsewhere in the Amazon. Or perhaps the malaria had become too debilitating.

No one knew for certain the extent or severity of malaria among that population. Garimpeiros were scattered in small bands throughout the Amazon Basin, testing their skill, luck and endurance. It was believed that at least half of them carried malaria parasites in their blood. The majority received no health care at all, and those who did medicated themselves with drugs they bought in town or from one another. A miner would typically visit a clinic only if he had become very ill; he would receive his medicine and take it long enough to relieve his symptoms. The most popular medicine then was quinine. But, as we already learned, the medicine was not completely satisfactory. Some of the parasites stayed in the victim's blood, rendering him a walking reservoir of the disease.

Evening was approaching and our group under the cashew

tree started to disband, for good reason. There were no lights on the unpaved landing strip, and Sister Irma had asked Sampaio for a lift back to Boa Vista. The FUNAI plane she was expecting had still not appeared. She had completed her mission and was ready to go home. Malaria transmission was waning. Besides, she was just recovering from an attack of malaria herself, and she had some kind of infection on her toe. She went to her hut to pick up the traditional Yanomami stone arrows she wanted to give to children in the south of Brazil. That was all of her luggage.

Vaccine Trials Planned

The next day Sampaio decided to visit an area we had just flown over, a particularly remote region near the banks of the Rio Apiau. He was preparing trials of an experimental vaccine for malaria developed by Dr. Ruth Nussenzweig of New York University.

Sampaio had selected 200 families, or about 1,200 individuals, from among the inhabitants of the region. He was taking blood samples to be tested for antibodies against malaria. The researchers wanted to know what antibodies people had in their blood before they received the experimental vaccine. "Then we can see," he said, "how much of a boost the vaccine may have given each person."

Clinic Visit

The frontier town of Mucajai was Sampaio's first stop. He was bringing new supplies of medicine with him for the SUCAM clinic there. Shortages handicapped many of the remote SUCAM clinics where the supply of antimalarial drugs did not keep up with the demand. Mucajai had 15,000 inhabitants, but officials had reported 2,882 cases of malaria in 1989, compared with 753 cases in 1987.[3] In other words, incidence of the disease had almost quadrupled here in only two years, and the local government-funded clinic had run out of medicine.

Sampaio also brought a new supply of vials for the serological or blood work he would do the following week in connection with the vaccine research. In the clinic's foyer he talked with a woman who was waiting to get the results from her new blood test. She had already finished the medicine for her bout with malaria several weeks earlier, but the symptoms had recurred, a familiar story in a region full of drug-resistant parasites.

Sampaio then settled down for a long talk with the local health inspector, Agios Lopez, who reported chronic shortages of many necessities, including petrol and DDT. Also, he said the malaria there was the worst that he had ever seen. The clinic at Mucajai was one of many SUCAM clinics throughout the Amazon that still used insecticides regularly — when they were available. Entomologists performing lab tests in the larger cities reported that the anophelines in the Amazon could still be controlled with insecticides. But epidemiologists and health workers in the field were convinced that mosquitoes here, like in other parts of the world, could develop resistance to any insecticide used against them. In many regions of the Amazon, especially in smaller, remote towns such as Mucajai, insecticides, effective or not, were often the only weapons available against the disease.

Malaria Doctor Makes Rounds

When outbreaks of malaria were particularly destructive in a given neighborhood, Lopez walked up and down the streets at dusk with his government-issued fogging machine, a device that looked like a hand-held rocket launcher. He was spraying a fog of mist on all the low bushes. He said he knew the treatment worked when he walked along the same route a few days later and didn't get any mosquito bites on his arms. Conversely, he knew the effects had worn off when the mosquitoes started biting him again. It was time to reapply the insecticide. The health inspector reported that he himself had had at least six bouts with malaria in the last twelve months. But he said that he always took his medicine right away and that he was never sick enough to miss a day's work. Apparently his acquired immunity combined with the medicine kept him on his feet.

Our last stop in Mucajai was the local hospital, staffed by two doctors from Boa Vista who took turns working 15-day shifts. Besides his job as physician to SUCAM in the big city of Manaus, Sampaio was a staff physician at the Tropical Hospital there. He was one of a small number of doctors in the Amazon with a specialty in malaria in addition to his specialization in tropical diseases. His wife was one of the few other doctors with similar qualifications. Sampaio was always eager to visit remote rural hospitals such as this one. Part of his responsibility was to bring the local health care staff up to date on recommended treatments and on the status of drug resistance. In return, he could pick up information from them about specific local characteristics of the epidemic and about new community-based plans for disease control.

A Good Place For Mosquitoes

As the road continued westward deeper into the hills, the forest thickened, parting only for a few sporadic isolated homesteads or for small streams with plank bridges over them. Sampaio said, "See that bridge? That's the one my wife and I and our co-workers had to rebuild after it was washed out. We had to build the bridge if we were going to be able to finish our job."

Sometimes when he came to that area he had a boat and a motorcycle tied to the top of his car. When a bridge was washed out he would cross the river by boat and continue his rounds on his motorcycle. Other times, if the river were shallow enough, the doctor and his team waded across. He showed me a photograph he had taken of his wife, two biochemists and a field inspector fording the river by foot, holding their medical supplies high above their heads to keep them dry. "This can be very unpleasant," he said, "because the *arraia* can bite your legs, and that is very painful."

Arraia was Portuguese for the stingray, which swiped its victims with its tail. Sampaio reported that the pain from such an attack could last up to 24 hours. But the perils and hardships were simply part of the job for the doctor and his staff. "Sometimes when the road is washed out we have to walk two hours to the last house and then walk back. Only SUCAM would go to this trouble to find their patients."

Our next stop was the health care outpost at the solar energy electric station. The SUCAM microscopist there said that a 3-month-old infant had died from *falciparum* malaria the previous week. It was the first reported death from malaria in that community in five months. The worker, Charles Miguel Bruster, appeared nervous talking with the doctor from Manaus. Bruster had been trained to recognize malaria parasites in a blood slide, to dispense medications, and to apply larvicide. He also was knowledgeable about everyone in the community. He said that incidence of malaria had increased locally after a new family moved there 10 months before. That family had moved from a region where the disease was so virulent that people were abandoning their homes. The newcomers had settled near the small river outside of town, a place where many folks came to bathe, wash their clothes, and play. Bruster said that after the child's death he had applied larvicide to the water near the bathing spot.

We drove up to the river, stopping first to visit an old man who lived near its banks. He had been very sick with falciparum malaria and still had a high fever. He was taking quinine, but it hadn't helped him — or maybe it had; at least he was still alive and able to get up out of his hammock to greet us. We asked if he knew how he had gotten infected. He said he didn't know, but he was certain it wasn't from mosquitoes. Offering his proof, he said while mosquitoes bit everyone in the area, not everyone got malaria. He cited as proof a 94-year old woman who lived nearby and who never had malaria, in spite of the bites.

We walked from the old man's house to the ledge overlooking the water. On the sand at a curve in the stream, a group of women washed their clothes with their babies playing at their feet. Two older children swung from vines over a still pool in the shade of the steep bank just beneath us. People have said that such pools were favorite breeding places for the predominant malaria vector in the Amazon, *Anopheles darlingi*. The female mosquito could locate blood meals and lay eggs all in the same neighborhood. She barely had to waste any energy traveling.

Boat Ride With a Volunteer

We drove a long way, sometimes as long as 30 minutes between houses, before we came to three houses in a small community at the end of the road. That was where the road met with and yielded to the Rio Apiau. Sampaio stopped at the house of a SUCAM volunteer, one of 40,000 or so residents who served as a relay point for blood slides or other supplies and messages and kept track of each person. This volunteer always knew when someone had a problem. If a sick person in a remote area did not show up for the results of his or her blood test, the volunteer would ride down the river to deliver the news.

Laurinda Rodrigues de Oliveira was a trader and the mother of three children. The doctor stressed how valuable she was to SUCAM. She sold kerosene and other items to the miners who came by boat to shop. She wasn't at home, so we walked down to the river's edge and found her fishing with her 3-year-old boy while her teenage daughter was scrubbing the family's laundry on a stone. In addition to her other chores, the daughter also helped her mother with the volunteer health care work. She went to school at the electric station and often delivered slides and messages to the SUCAM agent there.

Rodrigues said that her supply business was down sharply. She said 100 to 150 miners used to come in their boats every week to shop. Now, she said, very few came. But this didn't seem to worry her nearly so much as did the gravity of the malaria epidemic. There was malaria in every home, she said. It used to be all vivax malaria, but now it was mostly falciparum malaria. She told us about her own baby's malaria. She kept a respectful smile on her face and used a soft voice when she talked to the doctor. But she seemed to be shaking with rage. Her voice rose. She said her baby kept getting sick. He'd had malaria at least 10 times in the last two years. He would get his finger pricked for the blood test. They'd tell her it was positive again and give him medicine. He would get well for a month or so. Then the fever would return, and he would become very ill.

She paused to bait one of her son's fishing hooks with a small wad of moistened manioc, helped him cast his line over the water, and turned again to the doctor. She said that she had even taken her baby to the hospital for treatment. But in less than three weeks he was already sick again. It was falciparum malaria. Her voice became shrill, and she started to swing her arms as she talked. "I don't think this medicine is working!"

The two were quiet for a moment, with both of them hanging their heads. Rodrigues finally changed the subject. She had been a volunteer long enough to appreciate the realities of drug shortages and drug resistance. Renewing her composure, she started to tell the doctor about the other families in the area. One family had eight children, all of whom suffered from recurring malaria. Some families along the river could only tolerate the hardships for five or six months. They then abandoned their homesteads and went back to their former homes, taking their malaria with them.

The volunteer then invited us to join her in her boat to visit an Indian family badly stricken by the disease. With her hand on the throttle, she guided her motorized canoe through the dark water between walls of jungle so thick they blocked out the sky. Several kilometers upstream we reached the home the Indian family had carved out of the rain forest.

The path from the water's edge to the house was steeply uphill. It led over a low dike across a small swamp that looked as if it had been cleared for a crop, perhaps rice. Or maybe it was an enclosure for a turtle farm. Where the path swung around to the side of the house, a small open rainwater catchment had been dug in the ground. Banana trees and other vegetation were planted close to the dwelling. I began counting to myself all the places where mosquito larvae could be waiting to hatch.

Inside the house, everyone was sick — the parents and their five small children. The mother, Iris Moraes Gregorio, told a familiar story. They all had their fingers pricked by the health agent who came by boat. Her husband and the children tested positive, meaning they were infected by malaria parasites. Her own test was negative, but she said she still felt very sick.

The house was open on two sides, and its front faced the river. It was partially closed in the back where the husband stood on the sidelines. A baby slept in a hammock while two young ones — quiet with big, glassy eyes — sat on the floor by their mother. A vat for roasting manioc dominated the center of the room, and from the rafter hung the shell of an immense river turtle. The mother said that Rodrigues had brought her the turtle. The volunteer smiled and said the Indian woman was her friend. Then one of the older children, a boy who looked about 10 years old, came walking up the path with a shotgun over his shoulder. "He brings food for us," his mother said.

Jungle Musings

I started back to the river alone, for several reasons. I wanted to give the family some privacy while the doctor was there. They didn't seem embarrassed, but I was. I had no idea what a doctor could say to parents of children who kept taking medicine that was not making them well. But I did know he would be pointing out to them places around the house where standing water might be breeding sites for the mosquitoes that brought them malaria. I also needed a little privacy to restore my composure. I was not accustomed to seeing so many sick children.

At the side of the river, waiting for the others to come down the path, I was haunted again by the beauty and isolation of the jungle. One of the Indians had made a cage in the sand. It was a shallow square hole near the water's edge covered by a neat lattice of small sticks. I could imagine a newly hatched pet river creature living there until it was big enough to take care of itself.

I wanted to reach for some indistinct thoughts that had been following me ever since we stopped at the clearing in the river near the electric station. I thought about the age and perfection of the Amazon, and the age and perfection of the web of life we were trying to understand. The scene seemed familiar. It was as if this jungle had been here since the beginning of time, and so had I. Perhaps I had seen a picture of this in a children's nature book, the tangle of trees and vines with thick misshapen leaves heavy with moisture. If this were a picture from a book, there should be a dinosaur waiting at the next bend of the river. That's what the scene called for.

What if another huge disaster struck our planet and eliminated most animal life, like the event that wiped out the dinosaurs. Which creatures would survive? Probably protozoa, such as the malaria parasite. They are too wily to be extinguished. And they are too important. Would it be in the interests of the survival of the planet itself for the protozoa to survive to start a new round of evolution to establish new orders of creatures? New creatures for them to parasitize and new creatures to pollinate plant life and...?

Sampaio and the others started down the path to the river, and I put away my slightly intoxicating fragments of fancy. As we were beginning our good-byes at the river's edge, another canoe pulled up. It was Rodrigues' second canoe, with her daughter at the throttle. Her passenger was a SUCAM health agent from the clinic at the electric station, crisply uniformed with cap and satchel. He looked like an intruder in this jungle perfection. He unpacked his equipment on the bow of the boat and prepared to prick the mother's finger. First he cleaned her finger, using liquid from a bottle labeled "Revlon Nail Polish Remover." The doctor laughed. "It works just as well," he said. "When you run out of supplies you use whatever you can find."

Back in our canoe I noticed Rodrigues had a bandage wrapped around her own little finger. I asked what had happened. She told us a piranha had taken a bite. Was that the price one had to pay for capturing a river turtle? Not an unreasonable price, I thought.

River Stories

On the way back to the road's end, the volunteer and the doctor talked about the various dangers of the Amazon. She told the doctor three people had disappeared right here on this river, without anyone ever knowing what kind of creature took them. Sampaio said he also knew about mysterious disappearances on the river. He was born in the jungles of the state of Acre, the son of a rubber tapper.

His grandmother used to teach him lots of river lore, and he still loved to be on the river. He said while he was attending university, "I wanted to have a boat and go up the river and trade with people along the banks. It was a dream. Today I have 114 boats." He meant of course the SUCAM boats, indispensable to effective treatment of malaria in the Amazon.

Sampaio traveled the rivers whenever he could, to try to understand the Amazon, its people and their diseases. It took a lot of time. He said the more he learned, the more he needed to learn. He wanted to go up the Jarupa River, for example, "all the way from the beginning to the end. To visit all the little towns you would have to spend at least a month. Sometimes just to go from one house to another would take an hour or an hour and a half by boat."

His wife had asked him where he wanted them to go for their next vacation. He said he didn't see why they should go away: "I told her there are still places in the Amazon I haven't seen yet."

Malaria Hits the Cities

Malaria also was invading some of the cities of the Amazon. In the suburbs of Manaus, the inland river city of 1.2 million people, the disease was widespread. Mosquitoes were most numerous or most voracious where the jungle was being cleared to make room for the new residents from all parts of Brazil. They included the construction workers putting up new industries in the fast-growing city, road-building crews, discouraged settlers who could not earn a living on their new homesteads, farm laborers in the new orchards nearby, and the garimpeiros who settled on the fringes of the city while they sold their ore, rested and planned their next ventures. As the groups of newcomers mingled, so did the strains of disease they carried in their blood. Just like battle zones in wartime, Manaus was a malaria soup.

I toured the suburbs with the indefatigable Sampaio. We watched residents use shovels to deepen a gully behind the houses and clear vegetation from the stream banks. That allowed the water to move downhill quickly, eliminating any potential pools where mosquitoes could breed. It was an old strategy revived in places where medicines were not working well, where medical supplies were scarce, and where there never seemed to be enough doctors. In fact, the Tropical Disease Hospital in Manaus had to close its malaria ward because there were not enough doctors to staff it. The hospital staff saw their malaria patients in the ambulatory clinic and, if necessary, treated the critical ones in the laboratory.

Advice For Newcomers

At Brazil's Second International Symposium on Malaria in Manaus in October 1990, scientists discussed entomology, vaccine development and trials, and new treatment protocols. But the delegates were also concerned about designing new community-specific strategies with help from all the sectors of the affected regions. Attitudes about relying solely on high technology for malaria control were changing. Even "bench scientists" with a lifetime commitment to finding a universal cure for malaria were conceding that community-based strategies might be needed to try to hold back the disease until the new cures were available.

One of the nonscientists who shared the podium with the scientists and physicians was an American sociologist, Donald Sawyer, who was conducting research in environmental issues, and in human attitudes and behavior. He found that a variety of factors were related to the prevalence of malaria. Some social and cultural factors contributed to a high risk of malaria outbreaks, while other factors contributed to a higher degree of protection.

Specialists in the Amazon learned that in some regions most malaria was transmitted outdoors, in the daytime as well as in the evening. It had been known for a long time that some forest mosquitoes were quite active in the daytime. Indeed, the shadows of the forest canopy in the Amazon were often so thick that it looked like evening all day long.

Sociologists learned that most of the new settlers in the Amazon did not know how malaria was transmitted, and they did not realize that they themselves could take steps to provide at least a degree of protection for themselves and their families. Preliminary data showed that domestic animals around the homestead in deforested areas may improve a family's protection from disease-bearing mosquitoes, the way livestock kept in barns apparently helped protect farmers in the United States and Europe during the times when malaria was still endemic there.

Some Social Components

The need for new health strategies that combined the protocols of scientists and nonscientists alike was a theme expressed by the Rockefeller Foundation, which had a role in long-term projects for the prevention and control of malaria all over the world: "It has now been recognized that the purely technological approach to health has failed to produce the predicted improvements in health and well-being. One part of the failure lies in the incomplete coverage of the medical services actually delivered, but another part is due to the complexity of factors affecting susceptibility to and the ability to respond to illness. [...] What is clear is that the reduction of mortality has a major social component as well as a medical one. If we were to understand adequately the social component, and were to employ that knowledge effectively, then we might go far toward achieving the goal of good health for all" (Rockefeller Foundation, 1989).

I was curious. Could understanding the social components of malaria really reveal new ways to look at the underlying causes of infection and death from the disease? Take for instance the baby who died of malaria in his home on the Mucajai Road near the electric station. What were the social components? Did the baby die of malaria because his mother did the laundry at the river's edge at dusk? Because he did not eat enough protein to allow his immune system to function adequately? Because he had a case of measles, in addition to his malaria? Because his father planted banana trees close to the house allowing mosquitoes to breed in water collected in the leaves? Because his family could not afford mosquito nets? Because the road washed out, and his mother could not get him to the clinic for his medicine? The answers, of course, could not be found in the lab or anywhere. But understanding the questions might save other babies in the community.

Agriculture Policy Causes Malaria?

The state of Rondonia in Brazil's western Amazon was where the huge influx of settlers from the south were suffering the most. I visited hospitals in the cities, one of which was completely empty of patients due to a lack of doctors. I talked with health workers and researchers, and visited gold mining operations on the Rio Madeira.

In central Rondonia a new cassiterite mine reportedly was closed because of malaria and other problems. I toured the area with two SUCAM inspectors and a student helper. Driving south on route BR 364, we passed several long lumber trucks, one after another, carrying tree trunks newly cut from the rain forest. The road that took the trees out was the road that brought the waves of settlers into the western state of Rondonia. It was opened to traffic in 1965, and the "colonistas" started arriving almost immediately. The biggest rush of settlers started after 1984 when the new paved surface was completed as part of a large World Bank development project.

An estimated 10 to 12 million landless poor in south and central Brazil had been victims of the government's agriculture strategy, launched in the 1950s, which favored the mechanized production of export crops to replace traditional labor-intensive farming. They were casualties also of new industrial developments in the region. The idled farmers had two choices. They could join the ranks of unemployed in the slums of the big cities in the south, or they could migrate to the Amazon. The government tried to make it easy for them to choose the latter option.

An estimated 1 million new homesteaders came to Rondonia during the 1980s before the influx slowed. Government planners had underestimated the number of people who would settle in Rondonia and the magnitude of the problems they would face there. Once it began, there was no controlling the migration. The officially assigned plots were grabbed up fast. And nobody could control the settlers when they started clearing forests on their own. It became unofficial policy that anyone who cleared the land could occupy it.

Hardships Multiply

Hardship followed hardship. Most of the soil was nutrient-deficient, contrary to government brochures that promised immigrating farmers their own land with "a thick layer of humus accumulated during centuries." The jungle vegetation had leeched the soil, and once the trees were gone, very few soil nutrients remained for crop farming. Another hardship of course was malaria. Almost none of the settlers had acquired immunity to any of the Amazon strains of the disease. The World Bank took a lot of criticism for its role in developing and promoting Brazil's settlement schemes for Rondonia and the rest of the Amazon. The obvious defects cited were insufficient planning, unreliable research about soil conditions, and failure to anticipate possible health and social problems.

The malaria epidemic took the planners by surprise, but it could have been anticipated. According to specialists in disease control, people who planned big projects in underdeveloped tropical areas should always be ready for new outbreaks of malaria. It has happened before in other places, but never perhaps on such a grand scale. The World Bank president at the time, Barber Conable, admitted the mistakes in a speech in 1987. The Bank, he said, "misread the human, institutional and physical realities of the jungle and the frontier." The Bank subsequently collaborated with Brazil's Ministry of Health to develop and fund projects designed to address some of the new health and social issues.

Murder at Cassiterite Mine

Our car left BR 364 to take an unpaved road west toward Bon Futuro, and soon we passed through a settlement project called Alta Paradiso, or "high paradise," which boasted lush crops and pretty, well-kept farm houses. Perhaps Alta Paradiso had been built on one of the few pockets of good soil we had heard about. Close by we noticed the distinctive high-roofed, barn-like administrative buildings of the World Bank.

When we arrived at the entrance of the Bon Futuro cassiterite mine, it was obvious immediately that the place was far from closed. To one side of the entrance, a sluicing tower rose perhaps 30 meters high. Dump trucks were backing up the ramp one by one and unloading raw ore into the first of a series of sluices. The ore was shaken, washed and dropped to the next level for a repeat of the same process, and then down again until it was finally spewed out into a small hill of processed ore. Across the road from the mine, several small administrative buildings, including the main SUCAM clinic, were clustered. A large bundle lying close to the doorway of the clinic riveted our attention. The strange parcel was shaped like a six-foot-long cigar that was rolled in black canvas and tied securely. The gruesome reality dawned on us. That could only be a human body. Two mining agents came out of an office building to greet us. The men, an administrator and a geologist, represented a company that was bidding for a government concession to run the mine. We asked them to explain the body. "What body?" one of them said. He glanced at the rolled up bundle as if for the first time, explained that it was the body of a miner, and reassured us that a truck was coming soon to take it to the morgue. Gradually we learned a few details. The victim had been shot by a rival miner, who also had cut off the dead man's ear. No arrests had been made.

One of the SUCAM inspectors said that only 4,000 or so miners were still working at Bon Futuro and that the chronic violence associated with this group had started to abate. In recent months, there had been an average of only two murders a week, down from the average of four a week previously. Dr. Ana Escobar, whom we had met in Porto Velho, worked at the

SUCAM malaria clinic in the early days, when about 15,000 miners were there. She said the violence was so bad then it was hard to keep doctors on the job. Some doctors even quit to mine cassiterite for themselves. She recalled one day when a garimpeiro had approached her with his gun drawn, demanding malaria medicine: "You'd better take care of me now or I'll blow a hole through your head."

The mine was like a moonscape, with rolling vistas of denuded hills, large artificial, milky lakes, and twisted sand dunes. I couldn't make any sense of it. Heavy machinery was everywhere, trucks hauling away newly cut trees, large machines spewing river sediment on a newly formed dune, and earth removers of various kinds tearing away at the hillsides. A cassiterite mine was clearly one of the worst things that could happen to a rain forest.

We took a road around the rim of the mine, with the pristine rain forest to one side and the grotesque barren landscape to the other. We turned into the destroyed area and passed what seemed to be the largest of the artificial lakes. That was the location of the mine's first SUCAM clinic before it was flooded without warning by the mining authorities. We then reached an elevated commercial area in the middle of the mine, with disfigured hills and putrid ponds extending out on either side as far as we could see. After glancing at some of the shops, our first stop was at the new SUCAM clinic.

The agent in charge unlocked the door for the afternoon shift. Five or six miners were waiting on benches outside the clinic for blood tests to be taken or to be read. Before attending to any of them, however, the agent walked to the side of the clinic where a very sick miner lay on the ground in the grip of a typically violent malarial fit. He was helped inside for a blood test ahead of the others. We waited to see what the diagnosis would be. The miner was lucky. He had vivax malaria, and the available medicines would probably relieve his symptoms.

Then we traversed the moonscape to the largest barren hill of all. An earth remover was perched at a precarious angle near the top of the hill, slowly turning over new earth and shoveling it down the hillside. Several garimpeiros scurried behind the vehicle, some of them on all fours, with prospecting pans in their hands and bags of ore tied to their waists. Picking up small pieces of newly exposed ore, they scrambled and crawled all around the huge gyrating machine as it moved. It looked as though the miners were at risk of being scooped up themselves. We swung around and drove over the hill on another track. There, near the top of the denuded hill, were two big bright blue butterflies. I wondered if they would find a new forest canopy near by.

So Much Sidewalk

In the town of Ariquemes farther to the south, we remarked on the wide streets and expansive sidewalks. Sidewalks proliferated everywhere, even where there were no pedestrians or buildings. A work crew was laying out even more sidewalks as we drove along the main street looking for the Velerius Palace Hotel. In the empty clearing beyond our hotel, the wide boulevard and cement sidewalks wound out of town, reaching almost all the way to the jungle.

Ariquemes was a showcase for Brazil's plan to settle the Amazon with landless rural families from the south, but there was a wide gap between expectations and reality. For many of the migrants, the burdens of poor soil and malaria were more than they could endure. An uncounted number had been leaving, either heading north to Porto Velho or south and away from the Amazon for good. Highway BR 364, the new road that brought them here was taking some of them away, along with their malaria.

Some of those disappointed settlers returning to the south had reintroduced malaria to areas that had been free of the disease for 30 or more years. Several new cases of malaria, including ones caused by the *falciparum* parasites, had emerged in Rio de Janeiro, Sao Paulo, and other big southern cities. According to health authorities, practically all of the new cases had been traced back to Rondonia.

The new cases of drug-resistant malaria on the outskirts of Brazil's two most glamorous but congested cities were a shock to health authorities. So was the full-blown epidemic in Foz do Iguacu in the state of Parana, which was ignited by reverse migration from Rondonia. Many of the earliest colonistas in Rondonia had come from Parana, and they even gave one of their new settlements the sentimental name Ji Parana. That town, 365 kilometers south of Porto Velho on BR 364, was where the first outbreak of "frontier malaria" was reported in 1967. Incidence of the disease was still particularly high there in the late 1980s because the many mines in the area attracted so much rural labor.

Miners Avoid Treatment

Malaria among the miners was also keeping the incidence of the disease high in Ariquemes, according to the SUCAM inspector for the municipality, Regenealdo Batista Guedes. The problem reached emergency proportions after the discovery of cassiterite at Bon Futuro. The recalcitrant and sometimes violent behavior of the garimpeiros in Rondonia was as troubling to authorities there as it was in the state of Roraima, north of the Amazon. Many people believed the miners had the highest rates of infection, well over 50 percent, and by their own choice the least medical care. As was true of the smaller banks of garimpeiros in Yanomami country, the typical miner only took medicine when he was very sick, and even then he took only enough medicine to relieve the worst symptoms. They probably also had the highest mortality rates from malaria, but those figures had not been tabulated. As they zigzagged across the region, they carried with them a deadly cocktail of drug-resistant strains of the disease, leading doctors in Porto Velho to call them "descencadeadores da cadeia de transmissiao," or the openers of the box of transmission.

Malaria Capital of the World

There was a big difference in the way malaria affected the two most susceptible populations, the farmers and the miners. A miner would miss a day or two of work and then be at his garimpo, not perfectly well by any means but at least able to work. Conversely, malaria often hit the farmer at one of the two critical times in the growing season, either at planting time or harvest time. A short illness could make him lose a whole year's crop.

More than six out of every 10 people in Ariquemes had malaria in 1988, when this town of about 155,000 people acquired the sobriquet "Malaria Capital of the World." SUCAM records indicated that the incidence had dropped slightly in 1989 and 1990. Guedes was cautious, however, about relying completely on any figures on incidence of disease because of the many factors that could distort the numbers. SUCAM counted people who came to the clinic or who were visited by mobile health agents. People only came to the clinic when they were very sick and when they thought the clinic could help them. And the mobile health workers usually visited only homes in communities where they knew the incidence of malaria was high. Many sick people, of course, were never seen by SUCAM, or by any other health workers. Also, SUCAM had to cut back service in outlying regions because of shortages of petrol. Sick people in those areas wouldn't get their blood tests or be entered in the records. Some clinics had to give up service on weekends. If there were a shortage of drugs, people might have stopped going to the clinic altogether and medicated themselves with over-the-counter drugs from commercial pharmacies or with traditional remedies.

The health records, although not very accurate, were still valuable in terms of highlighting trends and producing raw data to be compiled in a new computer program being designed in Porto Velho. The program would analyze and compare disease rates over long periods in different regions, and discover statistically significant relationships among various sociological factors that related to disease prevention and control.

Guedes said SUCAM operations in Ariquemes were indeed being hurt by budget cuts. Health care workers were still being sent to the hardest hit areas, but sometimes staff had to buy their own petrol and forfeit their daily travel allowance. By late 1990, the clinics were also out of the drugs commonly used in combination with quinine. Such combinations, he said, were 95 percent effective against malaria in this area, while the cure rate for people taking quinine alone was minimal. But at least, he said, quinine was keeping most people alive. The death rate was low.

The number of settlers who had left Ariquemes was not available, but Guedes believed that more settlers were finally managing to overcome the problems that plagued them earlier and that more and more of them were staying on. One of the biggest early challenges for the colonistas had been cutting and clearing the forest, a task that often took several years. The more distance a farmer could place between the edge of the forest and his homestead, the safer he and his family would be from mosquitoes and malaria.

Guedes added that some settlers would eventually build up immunity to the parasite. And over the years they would be able to develop farming methods that would be better suited to their new homes. Nevertheless it was still too early in the history of the great Rondonia land rush to know if the city of Ariquemes would ever grow enough to fill its broad avenues and sidewalks.

Roadside Mosquito Nurseries

Brazilian doctors and researchers were trying to solve the puzzle of virulence of the *Anopheles darlingi*. The *darlingi* mosquitoes in the state of Rondonia were particularly dangerous, according to Dr. Agostinho Cruz Marques, director of the malaria division of the National Foundation of Health in Brasilia.

He said that 90 out of every 100 female *darlingi* in Rondonia carried malaria, compared with just 20 or 30 percent in the areas around Manaus. The well-known entomologist Dr. Wanderli Tadei, from the National Institute of Research in the Amazon, conducted a study of *darlingi* in the Ariquemes area and elsewhere, including the Tucurui Dam region in the state of Para. He found that the *darlingi* could change their behavior patterns quickly once they had left the jungle.

Scientists already knew that some mosquitoes, over a period of three to five years, could develop resistance to insecticides. The mosquitoes of the Amazon still seemed to be susceptible to the insecticides — at least for now. But indoor spraying didn't work because the *darlingi* typically stayed out of houses or at least away from the walls where the poison was sprayed. According to Tadei, they had made other behavioral changes quickly. Mosquitoes that had lived exclusively in the jungle before the settlers had cleared it were now thriving in the pastures and the low bushes surrounding many houses. In some places the *darlingi* that used to bite people only during the hour of dusk were now hunting all through the night, or even in broad daylight. Mosquitoes that had once laid eggs only in small pools of fresh, shaded water were now breeding in a wide variety of places around Ariquemes. Tadei's researchers found *darlingi* larvae in cattle watering troughs, on the leaves of fruit trees, and in pools created by fallen trees. They also found that *darlingi* were laying their eggs in the wide-open expanses of Tucurui Dam, allowing them to fill up immense areas of open water with their larvae, providing a larger and larger population of malaria vectors.

In Ariquemes, the mosquitoes were staying away from the city center, almost as if this were a rational choice. Tadei believed that they preferred an easy exit to the forest, at least in the early years of settlement. In a development proposal he recommended that new dwellings be located at least 1,000 to 1,500 meters from the forest. He also recommended that people create a barrier of thinned-out vegetation between the forest and the human settlements. A barrier of pastureland for dairy cattle might offer good mosquito protection, he said.

Dr. Marques also noted with surprise the ease with which the *darlingi* could take advantage of the new opportunities for breeding and feeding. Burrow pits or ditches along new roads in Rondonia were filling up with rainwater. The water could not drain because of a number of factors. The soils denuded of trees had weak porosity, and some of the drainage ditches under the new roads were too shallow, allowing vegetative debris to build up and to cause the drain-off from the rains to back up. All along BR 364 and the network of feeder roads built to welcome newcomers, the ditches were serving as roadside mosquito nurseries.

Ranchers Have the Best Land

Guedes suggested we drive out one of the feeder roads the following day to the town of Machadinho, a new settlement opened in 1983 as part of Brazil's big Amazon development project sponsored by the World Bank. Machadinho had since become a full-fledged municipality, complete with its own place in the record books, having probably surpassed Ariquemes at this point as the "Malaria Capital of the World."

That night, before going back to our rooms at the Velerius Palace, we noticed a campaign truck for Senator Olavo Pires parked in the back. He was a candidate for the run-off election for governor, and his name and slogans promising good health for everyone were widely displayed in Porto Velho. The next morning we were shocked to learn he had been assassinated the night before in front of his offices in Porto Velho.

The smooth unpaved road to Machadinho, 180 kilometers or so to the northwest, took us almost immediately into the rain forest. Soon well maintained ranches appeared between stretches of dense forest. There, as elsewhere, ranchers had the best land, close to the city. The ranchers had been here longer than either the miners or the farmers. They had more money, political experience and clout than the main bulk of rural colonistas from the south, and they had been able to clear the rain forest a long distance from their houses. There was not much debris of fallen trees left nearby where mosquitoes might find a pool of water for breeding. Most of the ranchers' houses had doors and windows and even porches in front. One ranch house sported a fresh coat of paint. Such luxuries were still out of reach for the newly arrived southern farmers.

As we traveled farther and farther away from Ariquemes we began to see some of the new settlements of the colonistas. Soon we could smell smoke. The road curved, and we saw a blanket of smoke that lay across the road. Some of the new settlers were burning trees on their land in preparation for planting. They were already late. The rains were due soon, and their first crop should already have been planted. Other farmers were tilling irregular patches of their fields in the low evening light, working around the charred, smoking logs and stumps.

We passed more small recently burned plots, most of them bordered on three sides by the rain forest. On each newly leveled plot there remained one or two very, very tall trees that the fires had missed completely. Often the solitary survivor was a sumauma tree, the tree that some Indians traditionally beat on to send messages a long distance. At one homestead, where skeletons of trees were still smoking, a pioneer family of two adults and two children was clearing patches of level ground for a late crop. It looked as if they would be able to plant less than one-tenth of their land. Could they feed a family of four with so small a crop? Their dwelling was a piece of that ubiquitous blue plastic sheeting stretched across a large fallen tree.

Brazil was not the first country to encourage its rural poor to tame remote wilderness areas and face unpredictable, almost devastating, hardships in the process. We remembered reading how pioneers in the U.S. Midwest had suffered through their own cruel trial by malaria. But the northern climate was on the side of the pioneers, who had the cold, malaria-free winters to regain their strength. Also, the topsoil in the U.S. Midwest was rich and deep, able to support crops year after year after year. One factor was the same in both places: the density of the swarms of mosquitoes.

The settlers of the Amazon had never seen mosquitoes like those. Some of them described dense clouds of mosquitoes that swooped down on them once the trees had been cleared. The sudden demolition of their environment had apparently driven away the various forest animals the mosquitoes had been using for their blood meals. But now new blood had arrived.

Frontier of the Amazon

Machadinho looked like a frontier town anywhere in the world, with lots of open space between sparse buildings. There was a clapboard hotel and a few small rickety shops, a huge petrol station with lumber trucks waiting in line for service, and a big open-air, screened-in restaurant where you could eat delicious food family-style, all you wanted for as long as it lasted. After unpacking at the hotel, our first stop was at the administrative buildings — designed in the familiar World Bank "style" — which housed the municipal, state and federal agencies. We talked to many workers there, but they were unable to provide us with precise answers to many of our questions.

The most difficult question was how many people lived in the municipality. Several people told us that the mayor would know, but he had left for Porto Velho to attend the funeral of the murdered senator. In the published reports we found a population estimate of 25,000 with more than half of them listed as infected with malaria in 1989. Another 1987 report indicated that 40 percent of the settler plots here had changed hands that year. We had already heard that not as many settlers had shown up here as had been anticipated. Our sources in the administrative offices explained some of the many problems that could account for the big turnover and diminished demand for plots. Most of the problems were variations of the same sad themes: poor crops and sickness.

Everyone confirmed that it was extremely difficult to make a living there on the land stripped from the forest. After a couple of years of farming, the crops began to fail. Government agriculture agents tried to encourage people to grow tree crops such as cocoa, rubber and coffee. Coffee was gaining in popularity, mainly because it was a crop with which many of the settlers had experience back home. However, the success rate, even with coffee, was not good. Most of the colonistas could not afford to wait several years before showing a profit, as they must with a tree crop such as coffee. For the great majority, as soon as they cleared their land, they needed to plant "survival crops" such as beans, rice and corn, to feed their families. Typically, they had to sell half of their land to speculators or ranchers to pay for seeds, farming implements, and chainsaws to clear more land. Some newcomers were forced to sell all their land to speculators. Such families usually stayed on the homestead as tenant farmers.

We asked the group of agents and officials if they advised colonistas to leave a mosquito barrier on their property, keeping their houses at least 1,000 meters from the edge of the forest. They said that was impossible for most of the poor, newly arrived settlers in Machadinho. The government workers were not sure that having livestock near one's house did indeed offer some protection from mosquitoes. But one man passed on some advice he had heard, a mixture of modern science and folk traditions. He said keeping a white cow in your field is good protection from malaria. Many settlers were buying one or two head of cattle — not for disease control, but as an economically viable way to use and conserve their land. The farmer could seed a pasture in two days with a minimum investment and then go away for short periods as need arose, allowing him more flexibility for off-farm labor.

Several discouraged farmers tried their luck at the garimpos, particularly the Bon Futuro mine, which we had just visited. They worked by the day on the lumber and construction crews. When they came back home, according to authorities in Machidinho, they often brought with them new strains of malaria from the other garimpeiros. Most of the group we talked to had come to the conclusion that malaria was here to stay. One person said that there would never be a cure for malaria because malaria was a "poor man's" disease. "If rich people got malaria, there would be a cure."

Malaria in Every House

Our conversation with the SUCAM Chief Inspector for Machadinho, Jaumir Marques Ferreira, did not offer a lot of optimism either. His problems were familiar — shortages of drugs and equipment, and high disease transmission rates. The inspector said that some charlatans in town were selling fake malaria medicine to desperate farmers. Because the supply of effective drugs was chronically low, the SUCAM control program was based almost exclusively on insecticides and on larvicides.

Ferreira said the malaria was particularly bad on certain roads in rural areas around Machadinho. On some stretches of road there was malaria in every house. He had mapped the houses in the high-risk areas, grouping them in "micro-zones" so he could schedule weekly visits to each one and conduct regular spraying or fogging programs. The death rate from malaria was not high. He estimated that there were 10 fatalities in the first nine months of 1990. A social worker had been hired to visit homesteads and to advise the new farmers on ways they could avoid mosquitoes. Mosquito nets and screens for windows were still too expensive for most of the people of this region, but draining mosquito breeding areas close to the farms sometimes helped.

311

The inspector was going out with a fogging crew that evening and asked us to join him. He also invited us to accompany him the following day on a tour of one of the roads where malaria was rampant.

On the way to the neighborhood where the fogging was to take place, we passed several boarded-up and abandoned houses. It was hard to know if they had ever been occupied. They certainly looked as if they had been empty a long time. We transferred to the SUCAM pickup truck, riding in the front seat while the SUCAM agents sat in back with their two fogging machines pointed behind us. As we drove slowly up and down the eight or so square blocks of streets, a thick white cloud of insecticide billowed across the sidewalks and over the bushes.

The health agents were using a Brazilian product that was believed to be much safer for humans than DDT or malathion. But still, the residents had not been warned that the fogging unit would be on duty that night. Several people out for a stroll saw the familiar truck and ran for cover. Others, including families with young children, walked unconcernedly through the clouds of toxic spray. One man in our wake was a local preacher on route to a prayer meeting up the street. He was the only person I had seen for a long time in a suit and tie. He increased his pace as the cloud enveloped him but managed to maintain his dignity.

In the early light of the following morning, the town had started to come to life. A lumber truck rattled out of town, and a she-donkey pulled a delivery cart up the street while a newborn colt wobbled behind her trying to keep up, his desiccated umbilical cord still swaying beneath him. Before long, Inspector Ferreira was escorting us north past an enormous lumberyard and down road No. 63, one of the many rural roads where malaria was very bad. Our first stop, a long way from town, was the two-room home of Aparecido Alves Pereira de Jesus, a former rubber tapper who worked as a tenant farmer on his brother-in-law's homestead. The health agents had painted the words "SUCAM 10" in large white letters on the doorstep of his dwelling, where he lived with his wife and their baby.

Pereira had planted a lot of trees around his house. There were coffee, banana, and rubber trees, and one large orange tree. Cotton bushes studded the landscape, and cats and pigs were everywhere. I tried to count the piglets that scampered around the compound, even squealing and running inside the house. But I stopped when I noticed a big pen beside the house that held still more of them. There must have been at least 100. The tenant farmer said the pigs were food for his family, but I was sure that most of them were destined for the market — assuming, that is, he had a way to get into town. He said that his first few coffee crops had been good, but that now, after five years, the yield was not worth picking. Next year he was going to switch to annual crops that he could sell in the marketplace.

His wife had recently been hospitalized, and she still looked weak. Pereira said he came down with malaria constantly, "500 cases in five years." The medicine distributed by the SUCAM workers only helped, he said, for a little while. Certainly 500 was not an accurate figure, but that must have been what it felt like for him.

His experience with malaria as a farmer here was certainly very different from what he saw as a tapper in the south. We asked him if he knew the location of the standing water where the malarial mosquitoes must be breeding. But he didn't think that was important. Many people had told him that malaria came from being close to water, but he still didn't believe it. When he was working full time in the rubber plantations around the southern city of Jaru, he was constantly close to water, but that didn't make him sick with malaria. Perhaps he had a mild case now and again, but the symptoms, he said, hadn't bothered him. But, in the north, the disease was taking a major toll, and the bouts seemed to be getting worse and worse.

313

The next stop down the same road No. 63 was "SUCAM 7," the home of Jose Baptista Almeida and his wife and seven children. They had migrated here from Cuiaba five years ago. Almeida said he had to work nonstop just to feed his family. There were a lot of coffee bushes and fruit trees growing around the compound, including papaya, pineapple, cocoa, guarana, and a black pepper bush. It occurred to me that perhaps the families who had settled here had brought the fruit-tree seedlings from their home regions. I could imagine hopeful colonistas, holding the young trees in their laps, as they rode the brightly painted buses north on the highways to their new homes, their hearts full of optimistic visions of the future.

Almeida said that he simply couldn't grow enough of the beans, rice and maize he needed to feed his family. His oldest son worked as a farm laborer for a neighbor so they would have at least some ready cash. The father was sure that the physical strain of his work on the farm was ruining his health. He had been hospitalized twice with what he believed were respiratory problems. But according to him, the doctors were unable to diagnose his condition. He put it simply and eloquently, "I'm not the man I used to be," adding that no one with a family as large as his should try to live in the new settlement areas. "People who come here are too poor. That's the kind of people malaria likes to attack the most." He couldn't even count the number of times he had been stricken with the illness during his five years in the Amazon.

He told us he still didn't have time to dig a well on his land. His wife and children had to tote their water in from a well down the road. He planned to take a gamble next year and to use one-third of his land for perennial crops — coffee and cotton — and to lay the rest up for a pasture for a neighboring rancher. It was obvious to us that it was a last-ditch effort, a far cry indeed from the hopeful dreams he came here with. If that last scheme didn't work, he intended to sell his land and relocate his family yet again.

Frontier School

Farther down the road we saw a Catholic church with open sides, a thatched roof and several rows of benches. It was a weekday, so the church was being used as a schoolhouse, and the benches were filled with children. Florsinha Alves Pereira de Jesus, the 25-year-old sister of the tenant farmer we had talked with two stops back, taught 18 children, ranging from seven to 14 years of age. She was born in Parana but had been raised in Paraguay. The teacher, who had only finished the fifth grade herself, was very proud of her children. She introduced each child and told us his or her grade.

When she heard our group was interested in malaria, she said the disease was "always present." She turned to the children: "How many students have had malaria in the last 20 days?" Eight children put up their hands. "I have to put up my hand, too," she said, "because I had malaria in the last 20 days also." She then asked, "How many have had malaria in the last year?" All but two raised their hands. We asked her if her students knew how one got malaria. The answer was clear: "Yes. If you live near water."

The teacher showed us the powdered milk-soy mixture supplied by the government for the students' lunch. Its label read "Nutricao e educacao constroem um pais saudavel," or "nutrition and education build a healthy country." "It's good for children to have this protein," she said, "because we can't even grow beans on this land." She showed us the school garden, with its pineapple, sugar cane and maize. She wanted to give me the only ripe pineapple in the whole garden, but I managed to stop her just in time before she cut the stalk.

As we stood in the garden, the teacher explained that the children who surrounded us all came from colonista farming families. The market for produce was very poor, however, and several of the children's fathers and big brothers had gone away to the rubber plantations to work as tappers, even some who had never tapped rubber before. All of the children walked to school along paths through the jungle. Some had to hike as far as four kilometers each way. The teacher told about the day two of the boys were late. When they finally arrived, they had a good excuse. The path they took to school went through the jungle. They were frightened by a jaguar and went back for their father, who brought them himself. "I think my children are very courageous," the teacher beamed.

Our final stop on road No. 63 was just a short way past the schoolhouse. Where the road dipped slightly we could see on the rise beyond that the hillside had been completely cleared of trees. The health workers got out of the truck to check for standing water on the side of the clearing. It was a variation of the same problem we had already seen several times along the roads of the Amazon. The bare hillside did not absorb the runoff, and rainwater was backed up in little pools alongside the road. We didn't have a cup to use to search for larvae. But Inspector Ferreira said that he had already examined the water on that stretch of the road. It contained *Anopheles* larvae, and he intended to return soon with the larvicide equipment.

Driving Home

The rain began again in misty drizzles as we drove back to Ariquemes. We passed a big lumber truck, shimmying a little on the hard-packed wet dirt road. The mammoth logs strained against the cables holding them. Soon we noticed a problem ahead. Traffic was stopped on either side of a dip in the road. We also pulled up to a slow stop, quite cautiously because the vehicle had begun to skid on the slippery surface.

My companions jumped out of the truck to investigate the problem. But I felt timid. The hour was approaching when mosquitoes can appear out of nowhere. Maybe this also was the hour when the jaguars started to get hungry. I reasoned I was safe from mosquitoes because the rain forest on either side of the road was untouched. Mosquitoes were probably getting their fill of blood from various forest animals.

Jaguars? I decided to trust my luck with them as well and got out to join my group down the road. I held on to the side of the lumber truck in front of us to keep my balance on the slick sloping road. Suddenly a loud eerie scream arose from the treetops. It must have been a howler monkey. These trucks and people probably seemed like a threat to its own territory.

Passing the trees in the truck, I hadn't realized how tall they were, but seeing them laid out horizontally in the lumber truck made them seem as long as a city block. I could then see the problem up ahead. Another lumber truck from the opposite direction had almost skidded off the plank-bridge at the bottom of the dip in the road. Two of its back wheels were hanging over the side. It did not seem dangerous, and it looked as if the truck would not tip over. Even if it did, the drop was only a few feet. But no more traffic would cross that narrow bridge that night until the truck was somehow moved.

Another lumber truck pulled up behind us, and another waited to cross the bridge from the other side. We all stood there in the soft rain and receding evening light while the driver of the lumber truck on our side unfastened the cable that bound his load of logs. He secured it to the front of the disabled truck. We backed up to give him room, and the driver retreated slowly, pulling the other truck free from the bridge. Then he secured his load again with the cable, and we all resumed our journey.

As we approached Ariquemes and night began to fall, I thought of all the children of the Amazon and the dangers they faced every day. They were all very courageous: the Indian boy hunting for food for his family; the volunteer's son casting his fishing line into waters full of threatening creatures; and the children walking to school along paths where jaguars lurked. Maybe this new generation would learn how to keep mosquitoes from breeding close to their homes. Maybe they would find a better way to treat malaria. Maybe they would find a way to live at peace with their world.

The End

---

[1] "The Amazon" refers colloquially to the entire Amazon River Basin, most of which lies in Brazil and some of which lies in Bolivia, Peru, Colombia and Venezuela. It is the largest drainage basin in the world.

[2] The chief source for metallic tin.

[3] Population for this city and all others in the Amazon are for the entire municipality, which includes far-reaching rural areas.

Bibliography

AAAS (1991). *Malaria and Development in Africa.* Washington, American Association for the Advancement of Science.

Ackerknecht, E. H. (1945). "Possible Factors for the Disappearance of Malaria from the Upper Mississippi Valley." *Bulletin of the History of Medicine*(Suppl. 4): 62-142.

Ackerknecht, E. H. (1992). *A Short History of Medicine.* Baltimore, Johns Hopkins University Press.

ACTMalaria (2000). WHO develops artesunate for emergency treatment of malaria.

African Business (2000). "New Anti-malarial Tests." *African Business* (April).

Agnew, N., et al. (1998). "Preserving the Laetoli Footprints." *Scientific American*(September): 44-55.

Agyepong, I. A. (1992). "Malaria: Ethnomedical Perceptions and Practice in an Adangbe Farming Community and Implications for Control." *Social Science and Medicine* 35: 131-137.

Ajaiyeoba, E. O., et al. (1999). "In vivo antimalarial activities of *Quassia amara* and *Quassia undulata* plant extracts in mice." *Journal of Ethnopharmacology* 67: 321-5.

Allen, S., et al. (1991). "Human Immunodeficiency Virus and Malaria in a Representative Sample of Childbearing Women in Kigali, Rwanda." *Journal of Infectious Diseases* 164: 67-71.

Alonso, P. L., et al. (1994). "Randomized Trial of Efficacy of SPf66 Vaccine Against *Plasmodium falciparum* Malaria in Children in Southern Tanzania." *The Lancet* 344: 1175-81.

Alonso, P. L., et al. (1995). "Authors' Reply to Letter by Trape and Rogier." *The Lancet* 345 (January 14): 135.

Alonso-Zaldivar, R. (2000). No title. *Los Angeles Times*.

Ambroise-Thomas, P. (1995). "Vers une vaccination centre le paludisme." *Rev Med Interne* 16: 717-723.

Andrews, J. M. (1941). General Considerations in Planning Malaria Control. *A Symposium on Human Malaria: With Special Reference to North America and the Caribbean Region*. F. R. Moulton. Lancaster, PA, Science Press Printing Co.

Andrews, J. M. (1948). "What's Happening to Malaria in the U.S.A.?" *American Journal of Public Health* 387: 31-42.

Andrews, J. M., and, Gilbertson, Wesley E. (1948). "Blueprint for Malaria Eradication in the United States." *Journal of the National Malaria Society*: 167-70.

Andrews, J. M., et al. (1950). "Malaria Eradication in the United States." *American Journal of Public Health* 40: 1405-1411.

Andrews, J. M. (1951). "Nation-Wide Malaria Eradication Projects in the Americas." *Journal of the National Malaria Society* 10: 99-123.

Arias, J. (1990). Interview with author.

Arnold, K., et al. (1990). "A Randomized Comparative Study of Artemisinin (*Qinghaosu*) Suppositories and Oral Quinine in Acute Falciparum Malaria." *Transactions of the Royal Society of Tropical Medicine and Hygiene* 84: 499-502.

ASTMH (1988). Abstracts of the 37th Annual Meeting. Washington, American Society of Tropical Medicine and Hygiene.

ASTMH, Ed. (1993). *Encyclopedia of Associations*. 28th Ed. Detroit, Gale Research Inc.

Babiker, H. A., et al. (1991). "Genetic Diversity of Plasmodium Faciparum in a Village in Eastern Sudan. Diversity of Enzymes, Proteins and Antigens." *Transactions of the Royal Society of Tropical Medicine and Hygiene*(85): 572-577.

Ballou, W. R. (1994). Interview with Author.

Balter, M. (1999). "Gene Sequencers Target Malaria Mosquito." *Science* 285(23 July): 508-509.

Banchereau, J., and, Steinman, Ralph M. (1998). "Dendritic Cells and the Control of Immunity." *Nature* 392(19 March): 245-251.

Banerji, D. (1999). "A Fundamental Shift in the Approach to International Health by WHO, UNICEF, and The World Bank: Instances of the Practice of "Intellectual Fascism" and Totalitarianism in Some Asian Countries." *International Journal of Health Services* 29(2): 227-259.

Bang, F. B. (1965). Malaria. *'Maxy-Rosenau Preventive Medicine and Public Health'*. P. E. Sartwell. New York, Appleton-Century-Crofts: 305-316.

Barber, M. A. (1929). "The History of Malaria in the United States." *Public Health Reports*, (October 25).

Barrett, O. N. J., and, Blohm, Raymond W. Jr. (1982). Malaria: The Clinical Disease. *General Medicine and Infectious Diseases. Internal Medicine in Vietnam*. A. J. Ognibene, and Barrett, O'Neill. Jr. Washington, Office of the Surgeon General and Center for Military History, U.S. Army. 2: 295-312.

Barrett, O. N. J. (1982). Malaria: Epidemiology. *General Medicine and Infectious Diseases. Internal Medicine in Vietnam*. A. J. Ognibene, and Barrett, O' Neill Jr. Washington, Office of the Surgeon General and Center for Military History, U. S. Army. 2.

Barry, M. (1992). Medical Considerations for International Travel with Infants and Older Children, Infectious Disease Clinic of North America: Health Issues of International Travelers.

Barry, M., and, Molyneux, Malcolm (1992). "Ethical Dilemmas in Malaria Drug and Vaccine Trials: A Bioethical Perspective." *Journal of Medical Ethics* 18: 189-192.

Bartzen, M. (1993). Interview with Author. San Diego, CA.

Barutwanayo, M., et al. (1991). "La Lutte Contre les Vecteurs du Paludisme dans le Cadre d'un Project de Development Rural au Burundi." *Annales de la Societe Belge de Medecine Tropicale* 71: 113-125.

Basco, L. K., et al. (1992). Chloroquine and Proguanil Prophylaxis in Travelers to Kenya. *The Lancet*: 63 (Responses to Barnes, The Lancet, 23 Nov. 1991, p.1383).

Bass, C. C. (1927). "The Passing Malaria." *New Orleans Medical and Surgical Journal* 79:10.

Bates, M. M. (1949). *The Natural History of Mosquitoes*. New York, MacMillan.

Bauxar, J. J. (1978). *History in the Illinois Area*. Washington, Smithsonian Institution.

BBC News Online (1999). "Mosquito!" *Horizon-Script*(October 15).

Beck, H., et al. (1997). "Analysis of Multiple *Plasmodium falciparum* Infections in Tanzanian Children during the Phase III Trial of the Malaria vaccine SPf66." *The Journal of Infectious Diseases* 175 (April): 921-6.

Behrens, R. L. (1992). Chloroquine and Prophylaxis in Travelers to Kenya. *The Lancet*: 63.

Bermejo, A., and, Veeken, H. (1992). Insecticide-Impregnated Bed Nets for Malaria Control: A Review of the Field Trials. *Bulletin of the World Health Organization*: 293-296.

Bernard, K. W., et al. (1989). "Epidemiological Surveillance in Peace Corps Volunteers: A Model for Monitoring Health in Temporary Residents of Developing Countries." *International Journal of Epidemiology* 18: 220-226.

Biggar, R. J., et al. (1981). Malaria, Sex, and Place of Resistance as Factors in Antibody Response to Epstein-Barr Virus in Ghana, West Africa. *The Lancet*: 115-118.

Bishop, E. L. (1934). "The TVA's New Deal in Health." *American Journal of Public Health* 24: 1023-7.

Bishop, E. L. (1937). "Consideration of Malaria Problem in the Tennessee Valley." *Southern Medical Journal* 30: 858-61.

Bishop, E. L., et al. (1948). "Malaria Control Trends on Impounded Waters of the Tennessee Valley." *Journal of the National Malaria Society* 7: 12-22.

Bispham, W. N. (1939). "Malaria in the Southern States." *Southern Medical Journal*(3.8): 848-851.

Blake, J. B. (1959). *Public Health in the Town of Boston 1630-1822.* Cambridge, Harvard University Press.

Blanton, R. E. (1991). "Still Hope for Malaria Vaccine," *Nature:* 199-200.

Board on Science and Technology for International Affairs and the Institute of Medicine (1987). *The U. S. Capacity to Address Tropical Infectious Disease Problems,* National Academy Press.

Bonair, A., et al. (1989). "Medical Technologies in Developing Countries: Issues of Technology Development, Transfer, Diffusion and Use." *Social Science and Medicine* 28: 69-81.

Borst, B. (1999). Malaria Resists Treatment and Cure. *The Boston Globe,* (October 25).

Bouman, H. (1990). Levels of DDT and Metabolites in Breast Milk from Kwa-Zulu Mothers after DDT Application for Malaria Control. *Bulletin of the World Health Organization.* 68.

Bourke, A. T. C., and, Joy, Robert (1967). "Malaria as Understood by Soldiers." *Millitary Medicine* 132: 366.

Boyd, M. F., Ed. (1941). *Historical Introduction to the Symposium on Malaria.* Symposium on Malaria: With Special Reference to North America and the Caribbean Region. Lancaster, PA, Science Press Printing Co.

Boyd, M. F. (1941). "An Historical Sketch of the Prevalence of Malaria in North America." *American Journal of Tropical Medicine* 21: 223-244.

Bradley, G. H., and, Fritz, R. F. (1946). "Entomological Evaluation of DDT Residual Spraying for Malaria Control." *Journal of the National Malaria Society* 5: 141-145.

Bradley, G. H. (1966). A Review of Malaria Control and Eradication in the United States. *Mosquito News.* 26: 462-470.

Bradley, D. J. (1989). "Current Trends in Malaria in Britain." *Journal of the Royal Society of Medicine* 82: 8-13.

Britannica, Encyclopedia (1965). Modern Slave Trade. 20: 20.

Britannica, Encyclopedia (1965). Portuguese East Africa. 18: 284-288.

Britannica, Encyclopedia (1965). Spanish-American War. 21: 149-151.

Britannica, Encyclopedia (1965). WW I. 23: 775.

Brooke, J. (1990). 'Is gold worth this? Amazon is being poisoned.' *New York Times* (August 2) A4.

Brooks, M. H. (1967). "Pathophysiology of Acute Falciparum Malaria." *American Journal of Medicine.* 735-750.

Brothwell, D. R., and, Sandison, A. T. (1967). *Disease in Antiquity.* Springfield, IL, C. C. Thomas.

Brown, E. R. (1960). *Rockefeller Medicine Men: Medicine and Capitalism in America.* Berkeley, University of California Press.

Brown, D. (1999). Malaria fight to focus on bed nets; 30-fold increase in Africa is urged. *Washington Post,* (October 13).

Bruce-Chwatt, L. J. (1951). Malaria in Nigeria. *Bulletin of the World Health Organization.* 4: 301-327.

Bruce-Chwatt, L. J. (1980). *Essential Malariology.* London, William Heineman Medical Books, Ltd.

Bruce-Chwatt, L. J., and, De Zulueta, Julian (1980). *The Rise and Fall of Malaria in Europe.* London, Oxford University Press.

Bruce-Chwatt, L. J. (1988). Worldwide Malaria Eradication: A Dream or Reality?, *World Health Organization,* (August).

Bruce-Chwatt, L. J. (1988). "Cinchona and its Alkaloids: 350 years." *New York State Journal of Medicine* 6: 318-322.

Brunetti, R., et al. (1954). "An Outbreak of Malaria in California, 1952-1953." *American Journal of Tropical Medicine and Hygiene* 3: 779-788.

Bruster, C. M. (1990). Interview with Author.

Bureau for Africa (1982). Manual on Malaria Control in Primary Health Care in Africa. Washington, *Agency for International Development.*

Burgner, D., and, Hickey, M. (1992). "Severity of Imported Falciparum Malaria." *British Medical Journal* 305: 957. Response to Stephen J. Lewis: "Severity of Imported Falciparum Malaria: Effect of Taking Antimalaria Prophylaxis" 305: 741-743

Burnett, V. (1996). Researchers in Conflict Over New Malaria Vaccine. *Seattle Post-Intelligencer,* (September 23), A4.

Busvine, J. R. (1956). "The Significance of Insecticide-Resistant Strains (With Special Reference to Pests of Medical Importance)." *Bulletin of the World Health Organization* 155: 389-401.

Buttinger, J. (1968). *Vietnam: A Political History.* New York, Praeger.

Camargo, L. M. (1990). Interview with Author.

Campbell, C. C. (1985). Interview with Author. Atlanta, Georgia.

Campbell, K. (1988). Refugees Health Symposium, In Association with 37th Annual Meeting of the American Society of Tropical Medicine and Hygiene. *Taped Presentation.* Washington, D.C.

Campbell, C. S. (1991). "Challenges Facing Antimalarial Therapy in Africa." *Journal of Infectious Diseases* 163: 1207-1211.

Canfield, C. (1969). 'Renal and Hematologic Complications of Acute Falciparum Malaria in Vietnam.' *Bulletin of the New York Academy of Medicine,* 45(10): 1043-57

Cannon, P. R., Ed. (1941). *Some Pathologic Aspects of Human Malaria.* Publication of the American Association for the Advancement of Science. Lancaster, PA, Science Press Printing Co.

Carlson, D. G. (1977). African Fever, Prophylactic, Quinine and Statistical Analysis: Factors in the European Penetration of Hostile West African Environment. *Bulletin of the History of Medicine.* 51: 386-396.

Carme, B. (1992). Pseudo-Resistant Malaria in Tropical Countries. *The Lancet.* 340(10 Oct.): 896-7

Carter, H. R. (1914). "Impounded Water: Some General Considerations on its Effect on the Prevalence of Malaria." *Public Health Reports* (Reprint No. 244).

Carter, H. R. (1919). "The Malaria Problem of the South." *Public Health Reports* 34(22 Aug.): 1927-35.

Cartwright, F. F. (1972). *Disease and History*. London, Hart Davis.

Cassidy, J. H. (1989). Medical Men and the Ecology of the Old South. *Science and Medicine in the Old South*. R. Numbers, and Savitt, Todd Lee. Baton Rouge, Louisiana State University Press.

Cattani, J. A. (1989). "Malaria Vaccines: Results of Human Trials and Directions of Current Research." *Experimental Parasitology* 68: 242-247.

Cau, H. D. (1976). "Rebuilding the health network." *World Health; A Magazine of the WHO* 34.

Celli, A. (1933). *The History of Malaria in the Roman Campagna*. London, John Bale, Sons and Danielsson.

Center for International Development (2000). Proceedings of the *International Workshop on Antibiotic Resistance: Global Policies and Options (Feb 28, 2000)*.

Centers for Disease Control (1995). *Malaria Surveillance,*.

Chanoff, D., and, Toai, Doan Van (1986). *Portrait of the Enemy*, Random House.

Charoenvit, Y., et al. (1991). "Inability of Malaria Vaccine to Induce Antibodies to a Protective Epitope Within Its Sequence." *Science* 251: 668-671.

Chen, L. C. (1988). "Ten Years After Alma Ata: Balancing Different Primary Health Care Strategies." *Tropical and Geographical Medicine* 40(July): S22-9.

Childs, S. J. R. (1940). *Malaria and Colonization in the Carolina Low Country, 1526-1696*, Brooklyn College.

Chougnet, C., et al. (1990). "Humoral and Cell-Mediated Immune Responses to the Plasmodium Falciparum Antigens PF155/Resa and CS Protein: Seasonal Variations in a Population Recently Re-exposed to Endemic Malaria." *American Journal of Tropical Medicine and Hygiene* 43(3): 234-242.

Churchill, D., et al. (1992). Chloroquine and Proguanil Prophylaxis in Travelers to Kenya. *The Lancet*. 63.

CHWA (1989). Mosquito-Transmitted Malaria in California: 1988-1989, Part 1. *California Morbidity.* 50/51.

CHWA (1990). Locally Acquired P. Vivax Malaria- San Diego County. *California Morbidity.* 27/28.

CHWA (1990). Mosquito-Transmitted Malaria in California: 1988-1989, Part 2. *California Morbidity.* 52.

Clark, I. (1992). *Tumor Necrosis Factors in Malaria.* New York, Raven Press.

Cleary, D. (1990). *Anatomy of the Amazon Gold Rush.* Iowa City, University of Iowa Press.

Cloudsley-Thompson, J. L. (1972). *Insects and History.* London, Hart Davis.

Coates, J. B., Jr., Ed. (1968). *Internal Medicine in World War II*, Office of the Surgeon General, Department of the Army.

Cockburn, A. (1963). *The Evolution and Eradication of Infectious Diseases.* Baltimore, MD, Johns Hopkins University Press.

Coggeshall, L. T. (1941). *Humoral Immunity in Malaria.* Lancaster, PA, Science Press Printing Co.

Cohen, M. N. (1989). *Health and the Rise of the Civilization.* New Haven ,CT, The Yale University Press.

Cohen, B. (1994). *The Vietnam Guidebook*, Houghton Mifflin Company.

Colbourne, M. (1966). *Malaria in Africa*, Oxford University Press.

Collins, W. E., et al. (1996). "Malaria vaccine [Letters to the Editor]." *The Lancet* 348(November 16): 1377.

Condon-Rall, M. E. (1991). "Allied Cooperation in Malaria Prevention and Control: The World War II Southwest Pacific Experience." *Journal of History of Medicine and Allied Sciences* 46: 493-513.

Cone (1979). *History of American Pediatrics*, Boston; Little, Brown.

Conlon, C. (1990). Imported Malaria. *The Practitioner* 234: 841-843.

Cook, G. C. (1989). "The Great Malaria Problem: Where is the Light at the End of the Tunnel?" *Journal of Infection* 18: 1-10.

Cook, G. C. (1990). *Parasitic Disease in Clinical Practice.* London, Springer-Verlag.

Cottingham, A. J., et al. (1966). A Prospective Study of Malaria Incidence Among Indigenous and U.S. Forces During Combat Operations, U. S. Army Medical Research Team.

Courval, J. M. (1993). *Estimating the Impact of Malaria Control on Mortality in Infants and Children,* Columbia University.

Couto, J. S., et al. (1991). Malaria Chemoprophylaxis with Mefloquine. *The Lancet:* 1479-1480.

Covell, S. G. (1967). "The Story of Malaria." *Journal of Tropical Medicine and Hygiene* 70: 281-285.

Cowper, L. (1985). Interview with Author. Washington, D.C.

Cox, F. E. G. (1991). "Variation and Vaccination". *Nature.* 349: 193.

Cox, F. E. G. (1991). "Which Way for Malaria?". *Nature.* 331: 486-487.

Cox, F. E. G. (1992). Malaria, Getting into the Liver. *Nature:* 361-362.

Craig, C. F. (1941). Cyclical Variations in the Incidence of Malaria. *A Symposium on Human Malaria: With Special Reference to North America and the Caribbean Region. Publication of the American Association for the Advancement of Science.* F. R. Moulton. Lancaster, PA, Science Press Printing Co.

Curtis, H. (1983). *Biology.* New York, Worth Publishers, Inc.

D'Alessandro, U., et al. (1995). "Efficacy Trial of Malaria Vaccine SPf66 in Gambian Infants." *The Lancet* 346(Aug 19): 462-467.

Davidson, B. (1987). 'Africa in Historical Perspectives.' *Africa South of the Sahara:* 3-16, Sixteenth Edition, Europa Publications Limited, London, England.

Davidson, G. (1982). Who Doesn't Want to Eradicate Malaria? *New Scientist,* (December 16).

Day, L. (1989). Immune System Seen Causing Malaria in Anemia. *University of California News Service,* (June 6).

de Oliveira, L. R. (1990). Interview with Author.

Derryberry, O. M. (1953). Health Conservation Activities of TVA.

Desouza, J. M. (1990). Interview with Author.

Desowitz, R. S. (1976). How the Wise Men Brought Malaria to Africa. *Natural History.* 85: 36-44.

Desowitz, R. S. (1991). *The Malaria Capers.* New York, W. W. Norton and Co.

Di Maggio, C., et al. (1991). "Malaria in an Urban Emergency Department: Epidemiology and Diagnostic Features of 25 Cases." *American Journal of Emergency Medicine* 9(4): 347-349.

Dirks, K. R. (1972). The U.S. Army Medical Research and Development Effort in the Southwest Asian Conflict. Washington, *Industrial College of the Armed Forces.*

Doane, N. L. (1985). *Indian Doctor Book.* Charlotte, NC, Doane, Nancy Locke.

Doolan, D. L., et al. (1998). "DNA Vaccination as an Approach to Malaria Control: Current Status and Strategies." *Current Topics in Microbiology and Immunology* 226: 37-56.

Doyle, E., et al. (1986). *The North — The Vietnam Experience,* Boston Publishing Co.

Duffy, J. (1979). *The Healers: A History of American Medicine.* Urbana, University of Illinois Press.

Duffy, J. (1992). *The Sanitarians: A History of American Public Health.* Urbana, University of Illinois Press.

Duran-Reynals, M. L. (1946). *The Fever Bark Tree.* London, W. H. Allen.

Durham, W. H. (1991). *Coevolution; Genes, Culture and Human Density.* Stanford, Stanford University Press.

Dutta, H., et al. (1978). "Malaria Ecology: A Global Perspective." *Social Science and Medicine* 12: 69-84.

Ebrahim, G. R. (1968). *Practical Maternal & Child Health Problems in Tropical Africa,* East African Literature Bureau.

Economist (1993). One Bite is One Too Many. *The Economist:* 33-4, (August 21).

Editorial (1991). Drawing the Curtain on Malaria. *The Lancet:* 1515.

Editorial (1992). "Malaria Prophylaxis." *East Africa Medical Journal* 69: 297.

Editorial (1992). "Rediscovering Wormwood: *Qinghaosu* for Malaria." *The Lancet*: 649.

Ehrlich, P. R. (1966). *The Machinery of Nature*. New York, Simon & Schuster.

Ellis, J. H. (1992). *Yellow Fever and Public Health in the New South*. Lexington, KY, University Press of Kentucky.

Elmendorf, J. J. (1941). *Malaria Survey — Methods and Procedures*. Lancaster, PA, Science Press Printing Co.

Encarta Encyclopedia Online (2000). Mozambique.

Engers, H. D., et al. (1996). Progress on Vaccines Against Parasites. *New Approaches to Stabilisation of Vaccine Potency*. F. Brown. 87: 73-84.

Erunkulu, O. A., et al. (1992). "Severe Malaria in Gambian Children is not due to a Lack of Previous Exposure to Malaria." *Clinical and Experimental Immunology* 89: 296-300.

Ettling, M. (1990). Malaria Clinics in Thailand. *The Magazine of the World Health Organization*.

Evans, H. (1989). European Malaria Policy in the 1920's and 1930's. *ISIS*. 80: 40-59.

Ewald, P. W. (1994). On Darwin, Snow, and Deadly Diseases. *Natural History*: 42-45.

Ezejie, G. C., et al. (1990). Malaria and its Treatment in Rural Villages of Aboh Mbaise, Imo State, Nigeria. *Acta Tropica*. 48: 17-24.

Fackelmann, K. (1999). Genetic Map Tracks Malaria. *U.S.A. Today*: D1, (November 2).

Faust, E. C. (1939). "What the Life Insurance Companies Think of Malaria." *Southern Medical Journal* 32: 689-693.

Faust, E. C. (1941). The Distribution of Malaria in North America, Mexico, and the West Indies. *A Sympoium on Human Malaria: With Special Reference to North America and the Caribbean Region*. F. R. Moulton. Lancaster, PA, Science Press Printing Co. 15: 8-18.

Faust, E. C. (1945). "Clinical and Public Health Aspects of Malaria in the United States from a Historical Perspective." *American Journal of Medicine* 25: 185-203.

Fauvet, P. (1999). "Mozambique's Foreign Debt." *BBC News Online* (June 3).

Feagin, J. E. (2000). *Electronic correspondence with author.*

Federal Ministry of Health, Nigeria. (1989). *Guidlines for Malaria Control in Nigeria.*

Ferrari, J. (1990). Interview with Author.

Ferreira, J. M. (1990). Interview with Author.

Ferrel, J. (1931). "Challenge of Malaria in the South." *American Journal of Public Health* 21: 355-376.

Fisher, G. U. (1970). "Malaria in Soldiers Returning from Vietnam: Epidemiologic,Therapeutic and Clinical Studies." *American Journal of Tropical Medicine and Hygiene* 19: 27-39.

Fleming, A. F. (1984). "Anaemia in Young Primigravidae in the Guinea Savanna of Nigeria: Sickle-Cell Trait Gives Partial Protection Against Malaria." *Annals of Tropical Medicine and Parasitology* 78: 395-404.

Fleming, A. F. (1989). "Tropical Obstetrics Gynaecology. Anaemia in Pregnancy in Tropical Africa." *Transactions of the Royal Society of Tropical Medicine and Hygiene* 83: 441-448.

Fox, R. M., et al. (1964). *Introduction to Comparative Entomology.* New York, Reinhold Pub. Corp.

Freedman, D. O. (1992). "Imported Malaria — Here to Stay." *American Journal of Medicine* 93: 239-242.

Fried, M., et al. (1998). "Maternal malaria and parasite adhesion." *Journal of Molecular Medicine* 76: 162-171.

Friedman, M. J., et al. (1981). The Biochemistry of Resistance to Malaria. *Scientific American,* (March).

Gabaldon, A. (1981). "Global Eradication of Malaria: Changes of Strategy and Future Outlook." *American Journal of Tropical Medicine and Hygiene* 18(5).

Gendrel, D., et al. (1992). When is Fever Malaria? *The Lancet.* 339: 691.

Gilles, H. M. (1989). "Malaria, an Overview." *Journal of Infection* 18: 1-23.

Gillespie, J. L. (1963). *Malaria and the Defense of Bataan.* Washington, U. S. Army.

Gillet, J. D. (1990). Forlorn Hope for Malaria Vaccine? *Nature.* 348: 494.

Gingrich, J. B., et al. (1990). "Hyperendemic Malaria in a Thai Dependence of Year-Round Transmission on Focal and Seasonally Circumscribed Mosquito (Diptera: Culicidae) Habitats." *Journal of Medical Entomology* 27: 1016-1026.

Ginsberg, M. e. a. (1991). "Mosquito Transmitted Malaria- California and Florida." 40(6): 106-108.

Ginsberg, M. M. (1993). Interview with Author. San Diego, CA.

Gish, O. (1992). "Malaria Eradication and the Selective Approach to Health Care: Some Lessons from Ethiopia." *International Journal of Health Services* 22(1): 179-192.

Gloyd, S. (1996). "NGOs and the "SAP"ing of Health Care in Rural Mozambique." *Hesperian Foundation News*(Spring): 1-8.

Godson, G. N. (1985). Molecular Approaches to Malaria Vaccines. *Scientific American,* (May).

Good, C. M., et al. (1979). The Interface of Dual Systems of Health Care in the Developing World: Toward Health Policy Initiatives in Africa. *Social Sciences and Medicine.* 13: 141-154.

Goodman, C. A., et. al. (1999). "Cost-effectiveness of malaria control in sub-Saharan Africa." *The Lancet* 354(9176): 378-85.

Gordeuk, V., et al. (1992). "Effect of Iron Chelation Therapy on Recovery from Deep Coma in Children with Cerebral Malaria." *New England Journal of Medicine* 32: 1473-1477.

Gosden, R. G. (1992). AIDS and Malaria Experiments. *Nature.* 355.

Greenberg, A. E., et al. (1990). "Mortality from Plasmodium Falciparum Malaria in Travelers from the United States, 1959 to 1987." *Annals of Internal Medicine* 113(326-327).

Griffitts, T. H. D. (1939). "Henry Rose Carter: The Scientist and the Man." *Southern Medical Journal* 32: 841-848.

Grmek, M. D. (1991). *Diseases in the Ancient Greek World.* Baltimore, MD, The Johns Hopkins University Press.

Grolier Encyclopedia Online (1993). DDT.

Guedes, R. B. (1990). Interview with Author.

Gunther, C. E. M. (1944). Practical Malaria Control. New York, Philosophical Library.

Hackett, L. W. (1941). Malaria and the Community. *A Symposium on Human Malaria: With Special Reference to North America and the Caribbean Region. Publication of the American Association for the Advancement of Science.* F. R. Moulton. Lancaster, PA, Science Press Printing Co. 15: 148-56.

Haggis, H. W. (1941). "Fundamental Errors in the Early History of Cinchona." *Bulletin of the History of Medicine* 10: 417-459, 568-592.

Hall, R. (1992). "Malaria Prevention." *Medical Journal of Australia* 156(103-105, 108).

Halpaap, B., et al. (1998). "Plasma Levels of Artesunate and Dihydroartemisinin in Children with *Plasmodium falciparum* Malaria in Gabon after Administration of 50-Milligram Artesunate Suppositories." *The American Journal of Tropical Medicine and Hygiene* 58(3): 365-368.

Halstead, S. B., et al., Ed. (1987). *Good Health at Low Cost (Proceedings of a Conference held in Bellagio, Italy, 1985),* The Rockefeller Foundation.

Haoll, T. F., et al. (1946). "Water Level Relationships of Plants in the Tennessee Valley with Particular Reference to Malaria Control." *Journal of the Tennessee Academy of Science* 21: 18-59.

Harinasuta, T., et al. (1982). "Recent Advances in Malaria with Special Reference to Southeast Asia." *Southeast Asian Journal of Tropical Medicine and Public Health* 13: 1-34.

Harrison, G. (1978). *Mosquitoes, Malaria and Man.* New York, Dutton.

Harvard School of Public Health (1994). *Health and Human Rights.*

Hayes, R. J., et al. (1992). "Case-Control Studies of Severe Malaria." *Journal of Tropical Medicine and Hygiene* 95: 157-166.

Hedstrom, R. C. (1997). "The Development of a Multivalent DNA Vaccine for Malaria." *Springer Seminars in Immunopathology* 19: 147-159.

Heineman, H. S. (1972). The Clinical Syndrome of Malaria in the United States. *Archives of Internal Medicine,* (April).

Heiser, V. G. (1932). "Discussion of Malaria Control and Anopheles Control Measures of the Past and Future." *Southern Medical Journal* 25(6): 651-655.

Hembree, S. C. (1980). "Malaria Among the Civilian Irregular Defense Group During the Vietnam Conflict: An Account of a Major Outbreak." *Military Medicine* 145: 751-756.

Henderson, D. A. (1997). "Edward Jenner's Vaccine." *Public Health Reports* 112(March/April): 116-121.

Herms, W. B., and Gray, Harold Farnsworth (1940). *Mosquito Control,* Oxford University Press.

Herrington, D, et al. (1991). "Successful Immunization of Humans with Irradiated Malaria Sporozoites: Humoral and Cellular Responses of the Protected Individuals." *American Journal of Tropical Medicine and Hygiene* 45(5): 539-547.

Hess, A. D., et al. (1945). "The Relation of Plants to Malaria Control of Impounded Waters with a Suggested Classification." *Journal of the National Malaria Society* 4: 20-46.

Hien, T. T., et al. (1991). "Comparative Effectiveness of Artemisinin Suppositories and Oral Quinine in Children with Acute falciparum Malaria." *Transactions of the Royal Society of Tropical Medicine and Hygiene* 85: 210-211.

Hien, T. T., et al. (1997). "Management of Multiple Drug-Resistant Malaria in Viet Nam." *Annals of Academy of Medicine* 26(5): 659-63.

Hinman, E. H. (1939). "Recent Advances in Entomological Knowledge of Malaria Control." *Southern Medical Journal* 32: 857-862.

Hinman, E. H. (1941). The Management of Water for Malaria Control. *Symposium on Human Malaria: With Special Reference to North America and the Caribbean Region.* F. R. Moulton. Lancaster, PA, Science Press Printing Co. 15: 324-32.

Hoffman, S. L. (1988 and 1991). Interview with Author. Bethesda, MD.

Hoffman, S. L. (1991). "Prevention of Malaria." *JAMA* 265 (398-399).

Hoffman, S. L. (1992). "Diagnosis, Treatment, and Prevention of Malaria." *Medical Clinics of North America* 76 (November): 1327-55.

Hogh, B. (1996). "Clinical and Parasitological Studies on Immunity to Plasmodium Falciparum Malarias in Children." *Scandinavian Journal of Infectious Diseases* Supplement 1 of 2: 1-3.

Hope, I. A., et al. (1984). Evidence for Immunological Cross-Reaction Between Sporozoites and Blood Stages of a Human Malaria Parasite. *Nature*: 191-194.

Howard, R. J. (1992). Asexual Deviants Take Over. *Nature*: 647-648.

Hsu, K. (1999). Drug Economics 101: Making Drugs, Profits and Doing Some Good. *The Boston Globe*: F1:4, (October 25).

Hsu, K. (2000). Biotechnology/Development. *Boston Globe*, (March 29).

Huffy, C. G., Ed. (1941). *Factors Influencing Infection of Anopheles with Malaria Parasites.* Symposium on Human Malaria: With Special Reference to North America and the Caribbean Region. Lancaster, PA, Science Press Printing Co.

Hunt, S. (1993). Interview with Author. San Diego, CA.

Hunter, D., et al. (1993). "Pesticide Residues and Breast Cancer: The Harvest of a Silent Spring?" *Journal of the National Cancer Institute* 85: 598-599.

Hyde, J. E. (1990). *Molecular Parasitology*, Van Nostrand Reinhold.

Inglis, B. (1965). *A History of Medicine.* Cleveland, OH, World Publishing.

Insect Control & Research Inc. (1983). AID Malaria Strategy Workshop (June 7-10, 1983), Columbia, Maryland, Agency for International Development.

Jaenike, J. (1994). Behind-the-Scenes Role of Parasites. *Natural History*: 46-48.

James, S. P., et al. (1932). "A Study of Induced Malignant Tertian Malaria." *Proceedings of the Royal Society of Medicine* 25 (May 5): 1153-86.

James, G. (1992). Mosquito Molecular Genetics: The Hands that Feed Bite Back. *Science.* 257: 37.

Jamison, D. T. (1987). *China's Health Care System: Policies, Organization, Inputs and Finance.* Good Health at Low Cost (Proceedings of a Conference held in Bellagio, Italy, 1985), The Rockefeller Foundation.

Jeffery, G. (1975). "Application of the Indirect Fluorescent Antibody Method in a Study of Malaria Endemicity in Mato Grosso, Brazil." *American Journal of Tropical Medicine and Hygiene* 24(3).

Jeffery, G. (1976). "Malaria Control in the Twentieth Century." *American Journal of Tropical Medicine and Hygiene* 25(3): 361-371.

Jeffery, G. (1990). Interview with Author. Atlanta, GA.

Jeffery, G. (1992). Unpublished Correspondence. Atlanta, GA.

Jekel, J. F. (1972). "Communicable Disease Control and Public Policy in the Seventies- Hot War or Peaceful Coexistence." *American Journal of Public Health* 62: 1578.

Johnson, L. W. (1991). "Preventive Therapy for Malaria." *AFP* 44(2): 471-478.

Jong, E. C. (1987). *The Travel and Tropical Medicine Manual.* Philadelphia, W. B. Saunders Co.

Joy, R. J. T., and Tigertt, William (1965-1966). Unpublished correspondence between Robert Joy and William Tigertt.

Joy, R. J. T. (1969). "Malaria Chemoprophylaxis with Di-amino, Di-phenyl Sulfone (DDS). I. Filed Trial with the 1st Brigade 1st Cavalry Division (AM)." *Military Medicine* 134(7): 497-501.

Joy, R. J. T., and Gardner, William (1969). "Malaria Chemoprophlaxis with Di-Amino, Di-Phenyl Sulfone (DDS). II. Field Trial with the 3rd Infantry Division." *Military Medicine* 134(7): 493-496.

Joy, R. J. T. (1990). Interview with Author. Bethesda, MD.

Kaker, P. A., et al., Ed. (1988). *Twelfth International Congress for Tropical Medicine and Malaria.* Amsterdam, 18-23 September.

Kar, S., et al. (1991). Duffy Blood Groups and Malaria in the Ao Nagas in Nagaland, India. *Human Heredity.* 41: 231-235.

Karbwang, J., et al. (1991). "Pharmacokinetics and Pharmacodynamics of Mefloquine in Thai Patients with Acute Falciparum Malaria." *Bulletin of the World Health Organization* 69: 207-212.

Karlen, A. (1984). *Napoleon's Glands and Other Ventures in Biohistory.* Boston, Little, Brown.

Karnow, S. (1983). *Vietnam, A History,* Penguin Books.

Keeney, E. B. (1989). *Unless Powerful Sick: Domestic Medicine in the Old South.* Baton Rouge, Louisiana State University Press.

Kidson, C. (1991). "Malaria Vaccines in the Future- What Strategies Now?" *Southeast Asian Journal of Tropical Medicine and Public Health* 22: 155-159.

Kiker, C. C. (1941). "Engineering in Malaria Control." *Southern Medical Journal* 34: 839-840.

Kiker, C. C. (1941). *Housing With Special Reference to Mosquito-Proofing for Malaria Control.* Lancaster, PA, Science Press Printing Co.

King, M. (1991). Malaria Control and the Demographic Trap. *The Lancet:* 1515.

King, M. (1991). *Letter to editor. The Lancet.* 338: 124.

Kirton, U. (1987). "Malaria, Agriculture and Development: Lessons From Past Campaigns." *International Journal of Health Services:* 17.

Klayman, D. L., *Head of Organic Chemistry Section, Division of Experimental Therapeutics, Walter Reed Army Institute of Research* (1985). Interview with Author. Bethesda, MD.

Klayman, D. L. (1985). "*Qingjaosu* (Artemisinin): Antimalaria Drug From China." *Science* (31 May): 1049-1055.

Kliks, M. M. (1990). Interview with Author. Ibadan, Nigeria.

Kliks, M. M. (1990). "Helminths as Heirlooms and Souvenirs: A Review of New-World Paleoparasitology." *Parasitology Today* 6(4): 93-100.

Kmietowicz, Z. (2000). "Control Malaria to Help Defeat Poverty, Says WHO." *British Medical Journal* 320(April 29): 1161.

Koella, J. C. (1991). On the Use of the Mathematical Models of Malaria Transmission. *Acta Tropica*. 49: 1-25.

Kovacik, C. F. (1978). Health Considerations and Town Growth in Colonial and Antebellum South Carolina. *Social Science and Medicine*. 12: 131-136.

Krogstad, D. J., et al. (1988). Antimalarial Agents: Specific Treatment Regimens. *Antimalarial Agents and Chemotherapy*: 957-961.

Krogstad, D. J. (1996). "Malaria as a Reemerging Disease." *Epidemiologic Reviews* 18(No. 1): 77-89.

Kuvin, S. (1992). AIDS and Malaria Experiments. *Nature*. 355: 305.

Kwiatkowski, D., et al. (1991). Bed nets and malaria. *The Lancet*. 338: 1499.

Kwiatkowski, D., and Marsh, Kevin (1997). "Development of a malaria vaccine." *The Lancet* 350(December 6): 1696-701.

Lackritz, E. M., et al. (1991). "Imported Plasmodium Falciparum on a Holiday Trip?" *European Journal of Clinical Microbiology and Infectious Diseases* 9: 910-911.

Lal, A. A., and Collins, William E. (1996). "Malaria Vaccine." *The Lancet* 348(November 16): 1377.

Lal, A. A. (1999-2000). Electronic Correspondence with Author.

Langer, W. L., Ed. (1980). *An Encyclopedia of World History*. Boston, MA, Houghton Mifflin Company.

Langmuir, A. D. (1963). "The Surveillance of Communicable Diseases of National Importance." *New England Journal of Medicine*. 182-192.

Lanning, M. L., et al. (1992). *Inside the VC and NVA*, Fawcett Columbine.

Larkin, G. L., et al. (1991). "Congenital Malaria in a Hyperendemic Area." *American Journal of Tropical Medicine and Hygiene* 45: 587-592.

Larrea, O. (1990). Interview with Author.

Learmonth, A. (1988). *Disease Ecology*. New York, Basil Blackwell.

Lederberg, J., et al. (1992). *Emerging Infections, Microbial Threats to Health in the United States*. Washington, National Academy Press.

Legters, L. J., et al. (1965). Apparent Refractoriness to Chloroquine, Pyrimethamine and Quinine in Strains of Plasmodium Falciparum form Vietnam. *Military Medicine.* 130: 168-176.

Legters, L. J. (1990). Interview with Author. Bethesda, MD.

Legum, C. (1999). *Africa Since Independence.* Bloomington, IN, Indiana University Press.

Lengeler, C., et al. (1996). "From efficacy to effectiveness: Insecticide-treated bed nets in Africa." *Bulletin of World Health Organization* 74(May-June): 325-8.

Leprince, J. A. (1932). "Malaria Control and Anopheles Control Measures of the Past and Future." *Southern Medical Journal* 25: 651-653.

Levine, N. D. (1964). *Malaria in the Interior Valley of North America by Daniel Drake(1850); A Selection.* Urbana, University of Illinois Press.

Lewis, S. J., et al. (1992). "Severity of Imported Falciparum Malaria: Effects of Taking Antimalaria Prophylaxis." *British Medical Journal* 305: 741-743.

Liese, B. (1989). Interview with Author. Washington D.C.

Lobel, H. O. (1989). Malaria and Use of Prevention Measures Among United States Travelers. *Travel Medicine.* R. A. Steffen, et al. Berlin, Springer Verlag.

Lobel, H. O., et al. (1991). "Effectiveness and Tolerance of Long-Term Malaria Prophylaxis with Mefloquine." *JAMA* 265: 361-364.

Lonergan, G. (1991). 'Malaria, Mefloquine, Madness, and Mosquito Nets,' *Letter to the Editor, JAMA* 265; 21(June 5).

Lopes, A. (1990). Interview with Author.

Lopez-Antunano, F. J. (1990). Interview with Author.

Lueck, S. (2000). Study Urges Rise in Spending to Fight Malaria. *Wall Street Journal:* A2, (April 25).

Luiz, J. (1990). Interview with Author.

Lwin, M. (1991). "Trial of Antimalaria Potential of Extracts of Artemisia Annua Grown in Myanmar." *Transaction of the Royal Society of Tropical Medicine and Hygiene* 85: 449.

Lyimo, E. E., et al. (1991). Trials of Pyrethroid Impregnated Bednets in an Area of Tanzania Holoendemic for Malaria. Part 3: Effects on the Prevalence of Malaria Parasitaemia and Fever. *Acta Tropica.* 49: 157-163.

Macdonald, G. (1957). *The Epidemiology and Control of Malaria.* London, Oxford University Press.

Mackie, T., et al. (1945). *A Manual of Tropical Medicine.* Philadelphia, W. B. Sanders Co.

Maclear, M. (1981). *The Ten Thousand Day War,* Avon Books, Division of Hearst Corp.

Maldonado, Y. A., et al. (1990). "Transmission of *Plasmodium vivax* Malaria in San Diego County, California, 1986." *American Journal of Tropical Medicine and Hygiene* 42(1): 3-9.

Mann, J. (1999). Leading the Effort Against Malaria. *The Washington Post,* (October 25).

Manning, A. (2000). A Better Life: Health, Education and Science. *U.S.A. Today:* 7D, (April 25).

Marques, A. C. (1988). Main Malaria Situations in the Brazilian Amazon Region. Brasilia, TDR/WHO.

Marques, A. C. (1990). Interview with Author.

Marsh, K., et al. (1996). "The Pathogenesis of Severe Malaria in African Children." *Annals of Tropical Medicine and Parasitology* 90(4): 395-402.

Marsh, K., and Snow, Robert W. (1997). "30 Years of Science and Technology: The Example of Malaria." *The Lancet* 349(suppl. III): 1-2.

Marshall, E. (1992). "Malaria Vaccine on Trial at Last?" *Science* 255(28 Feb): 1063-64.

Marti-Ibanez, F. (1961). *A Prelude to Medical History.* New York, MD Publications.

Matheson, R. (1941). *The Role of Anophelines in the Epidemiology of Malaria.* Lancaster, PA, Science Press Printing Co.

Matola, Y. G., et al. (1984). "Malaria in the Islands of Zanzibar and Pemba 11 Years after the Suspension of a Malaria Eradication Programme." *Central African Journal of Medicine:* 91-4.

Maugh, T. H. I. (1977). "Malaria: Resurgence in Research Brightens Prospects." *Science* 196.

Maurice, J. (1995). "Malaria Vaccine Raises a Dilemma." *Science* 267(20 January,): 320-323.

Maxcy, K. (1923). The Distribution of Malaria in the United States as Indicated by Mortality Reports. *Public Health Reports*.

May, J. M. (1961). *Studies in Disease Ecology*. New York, Hafner.

McCutchan, T. F. (1984). "Evolutionary Relatedness of Plasmodium Species as Determined by the Structure of DNA." *Science*(20): 808-11.

McKenna, M. A. J. (2000). "Africa Seeks 'Partners' in Fighting Malaria, AIDS." *The Atlanta Constitution*(April 14): A6.

McKeown, T. (1988). *The Origin of Human Disease*, Basil Blackwell.

McNeil Jr., D. G. (2000). Study Says Combating Malaria Would Cost Little. *New York Times*: A.10, (April 25).

McNeill, W. H. (1977). *Plagues and Peoples*. Garden City, N. Y., Anchor Books.

Mertz, K., et al. (1991). "Imported Malaria Associated with Malariotherapy of Lyme Disease." *JAMA*(16, Jan.).

Miller, L. H., et al. (1984). "Perspectives for Malaria Vaccination." *Philosophical Transactions of the Royal Society of London* 307: 99-115.

Miller, K., D. (1989). "Treatment of Severe Malaria in the United States with a Continuous Infusion of Quinidine Glucose and Exchange Transfusion." *New England Journal of Medicine* 321(13 July): 65-7

Miller, L. H. (1992). "The Challenge of Malaria." *Science* 257(3 July): 36-7

Miller, L. H., et al. (1994). "Malaria Pathogenesis." *Science* 264(24 June): 1878-1883.

Miller, L. H., and Hoffman, Stephen L. (1998). "Research Toward Vaccines Against Malaria." *Natural Medicine Vaccine Supplement* 4(5): 520-524.

Millikan, B. (1990). *Tropical Deforestation, Land Degradation and Society: Lessons from Rondonia*, University of California.

Millikan, B. (1990). Interview with Author. Rondonia, Brazil.

Mitchison, A. (1993). "Will We Survive?" *Scientific American* (September): 136-144.

Mizrahi, M. (1993). "Interview with Author."

MMWR (1999). SS-1(48): 1-23.

Molineaux, L., et al. (1980). The Garki Project. Geneva, *World Health Organization*.

Moore, D. V., and Lanier, J. E. (1961). "Observations on 2 Plasmodium Falciparum Infections with Abnormal Response to Chloroquine." *American Journal of Tropical Medicine and Hygiene* 10: 5-9.

Moore, P. (1993). Mortality Rates in Displaced and Resident Populations of Central Somalia During the 1992 Famine. *The Lancet.* 341: 936.

Moreland, S. C. H. (1991). "Malaria and International Air Travel." *Journal of the Royal Society of Health* 111: 21-3.

Moulton, F. R., Ed. (1941). *A Symposium on Human Malaria: With Special Reference to North America and the Caribbean Region.* Publication of the AAAS No. 15. Lancaster, PA, Science Press Printing Co.

Mountin, N. J. (1944). "Program for the Eradication of Malaria." *Journal of National Malaria Society* 3: 69-73.

Msuya, F. H. M., et al. (1991). "Trials of Pyrethroid Impregnated Bednets in an Area of Tanzania Holoendemic for Malaria. Part 4: Effects of Incidence of Malaria Infection." *Acta Tropica* 49: 165-71.

Muchie, J. (1986). Interview with Author. Washington, D.C.

Muraleedharan, V. R., et al. (1992). "Anti-Malaria Policy in the Madras Presidency: An Overview of the Early Decades of the Twentieth Century." *Medical History*: 290-305.

N'Gombe, J. (1985-6). Epidemiology and Control of Malaria in Warm Climate Countries. Livingston, Zambia, The Government of Zambia.

Najera, J. A., et al. (1985). "Social Epidemiology of Malaria." *Epidemiological Bulletin* 5(5-11).

Najera, J. A. (1989). "Malaria and the Work of WHO." *Bulletin of World Health Organization* 67(3): 229-43.

Najera, J. A., et al. (1992). Malaria: New Patterns and Perspectives. Washington, *World Bank.*

Najera, J. A., et al. (1996). The Burden of Malaria, *World Health Organization-Malaria Unit.*

Najera, J. A. (No Date). Malaria Control is Possible. *Public Health, No. 11, Main Theme: Malaria.* Bayer: 15-20.

Nathwani, D. (1992). "Malaria in Aberdeen: An Audit of 110 Patients Admitted Between 1980-1991." *Scottish Medical Journal* 37(4): 106-10.

National Research Council and Institute of Medicine (1987). *The U.S. Capacity to Address Tropical Infectious Disease Problems.* Washington, National Academy of Sciences.

Neel, S. M. (1973). Medical Support of the U.S. Army in Vietnam, 1965-70. Washington, Department of the Army.

Nelson, E. E. (1941). *Cinchona and its Alkaloids in the Treatment of Malaria.* Lancaster, PA, Science Press Printing Co.

New York Times (1942). "Troops on Bataan Routed by Malaria." (April 18): 5.

Ngatake, T., et al. (1992). "Pathology of Falciparum Malaria in Vietnam." *American Journal of Tropical Medicine and Hygiene* 47: 259-64.

Nicholas, J. B. (1942). Recent Mortality from Malaria in the United States, *Virginia Medical Monthly* (69).

Nicoll, F. (1999). "Q & A: Dropping the Debt." *BBC News Online*(June 2).

Nossal, G., J. V. (1993). Life, Death and the Immune System. *Scientific American:* 53-62.

Nosten, F., et al. (1997). "Phase I Trial of the SPf66 Malaria Vaccine in a Malaria-Experienced Population in Southeast Asia." *The American Journal of Tropical Medicine and Hygiene* 56(5): 526-532.

Nowosiksky, T. (1967). "The Epidemic Curve of Plasmodium Falciparum Malaria in a Non-immune Population; American Troops in Vietnam, 1965 and 1966." *American Journal of Epidemiology* 86: 461-67.

Nuland, S. (1988). *Doctors: The Biography of Medicine.* New York, Random House.

Nussenzweig, V., and Nussenzweig, Ruth S. (1990). "Progress Toward a Malaria Vaccine." *Hospital Practice*(September 15): 45-57.

Nussenzweig, R. S., and Long, Carole A. (1994). "Malaria Vaccines: Multiple Targets." *Science* 265(2 September): 1381-2.

Oaks, S. C. J. e. a., Ed. (1991). *Malaria, Obstacles and Opportunities,* Institute of Medicine.

Ochert, A. (1999). "New Wrinkle in Bednet Debate." *Science*(8 March).

Oduola, A. (1988, 1990). Interview with Author. Washington, and Ibadan, Nigeria.

Ognibene, A. J., and Conte, Nicholas F. (1982). Malaria: Chemotherapy. *General Medicine and Infectioius Diseases. Internal Medicine in Vietnam, Vol. 2.* A. J. Ognibene, and Barrett, O' Neill Jr., Office of the Surgeon General and Center for Military History.

Ognibene, A. J., and Barrett, O' Neill Jr. (1982). *General Medicine and Infectious Diseases. Internal Medicine in Vietnam, Vol. 2.* Washington, Office of the Surgeon General and Center for Military History.

Ognibene, A. J., and Barrett, O'Neill Jr. (1982). Malaria: Introduction and Background. *General Medicine and Infectious Diseases. Internal Medicine in Vietnam, Vol. 2.* A. J. Ognibene, and Barrett, O' Neill Jr. Washington, Office of the Surgeon General and Center for Military History.

Ogutu, R. O., et al. (1992). "The Effect of Participatory School Health Programme on the Control of Malaria." *East African Medical Journal* 69: 298-302.

Okanurak, et al. (1991). "The Role of Folk Healers in the Malaria Volunteer Program in Thailand." *Southeast Asian Journal Of Medicine and Public Hygiene* 22: 57-64.

Okonofua, F. E., et al. (1992). "Influence of Socioeconomic Factors on the Treatment and Prevention of Malaria in Pregnant and Non-Pregnant Adolescent Girls in Nigeria." *Journal of Tropical Medicine and Hygiene* 95: 309-15.

Olivar, M., et al. (1991). "Presumptive Diagnosis of Malaria Results in a Significant Risk of Mistreatment of Children in Urban Sahel." *Transactions of the Royal Society of Tropical Medicine and Hygiene* 85: 729-30.

Oliveira-Ferreira, J., et al. (1992). "Low Frequency of Anti-Plasmodium Falciparum Circumsporozoite Repeat Antibodies and Rate of High Malaria Transmission in Endemic Areas of Rondonia State in Northwestern Brazil." *American Journal of Tropical Medicine and Hygiene* 46(6): 720-26.

Olpes, A. (1990). Interview with Author.

Ortiz de Montellano, B. R. (1990). *Malaria in the South Before Civil War.*

Oswald, G., and Lawrence, E. P. (1990). Runway Malaria. *The Lancet*: 1537.

PAHO (1986). *Malaria Control in the Americas: A Critical Analysis.* Washington, Pan American Health Organization.

PAHO (1988). *Status of Malaria Programs in the Americas.* Washington, Pan American Health Organization.

Pampana, E. J. (1948). *Malaria as a Problem for the World Health Organization.* International Congresses on Tropical Medicine and Malaria, Washington, U.S. Government Printing Office.

Pasvol, G., et al. (1991). "Quinine Treatment of Severe Falciparum Malaria in African Children: A Randomized Comparison of Three Regimens." *American Journal of Tropical Medicine and Hygiene* 45: 702-13.

Patterson, C. (1978). *Evolution.* Ithaca, NY, The Cornell University Press.

Patterson, K. D. (1989). Disease Environment of the Antebellum South. *Science and Medicine in the Old South.* R. L. Numbers, and Savitt, Todd Lee, Louisiana State University Press: 152-165.

Paul, W. E. (1993). "Infectious Diseases and the Immune System." *Scientific American*(September): 91-97.

Perkins, J. H. (1982). *Insects, Experts and the Insecticide Crisis.* New York, Plenum Press.

Perrin, L. H., et al. (1988). Development of Malaria Vaccines. *Tropical and Geographical Medicine.* S6-S21.

Peters, D. H., and Gray, Ronald H. (1992). "When is Fever Malaria?" *The Lancet* 339: 690.

Petersen, E., et al. (1990). "Malaria Chemoprophylaxis: Why Mefloquine?" *The Lancet* 336(Sept. 29): 811.

Phillips, M. A. (1991). "The Operational Costs of Spraying Residual Insecticides: A Case Study from Nepal." *American Journal of Tropical Medicine and Hygiene* 44: 130-39.

Pividal, J., et al. (1992). "Efficacy of Dapsone with Pyrimethamine (Maloprim) for Malaria Prophylaxis in Maputo, Mozambique." *East African Medical Journal* 69: 303-305.

Pons, S. (1999). "Drug-resistant malaria lashes Africa." *Agence France Press*(March 19).

Powell, R. D., and Tigertt, William D. (1968). "Drug Resistance of Parasites Causing Human Malaria." *Annual Review of Medicine* 19: 81-120.

Prothero, R. M. (1965). *Migrants and Malaria.* New York, Longmans.

Prothero, R. M. (1977). "Disease and Mobility: A Neglected Factor in Epidemiology." *International Journal of Epidemiology* 6: 259-67.

Pursell, J. (2000). Unpublished research.

Raccurt, C. P., et al. (1991). "Imported Cases of Malaria in Bordeaux: Evaluating the Risk of Falciparum Infection According to the Country Visited." *Bulletin of the World Health Organization* 69: 85-91.

Raeburn, P. (1993). DDT Exposure Linked to Breast Cancer in Women. *Seattle Post-Intelligencer.* Seattle: A3 (April 21).

Ramos, A. M. (1990). Interview with Author.

Ransome-Kuti, O. (1995). Interview with Author. Washington, D.C.

Rapport, S., and Wright, Helen (1961). *Great Adventures in Medicine*. New York, Dial Press.

Rauber, I. G. M. (190). Interview with Author.

Ravaonjanahary, C. (1991). "The Impact of Anti-Vector." *Annales de la Society Belge de Medicine Tropicale* 71(1): 96-101.

Rawley, J. A. (1981). *The Transatlantic Slave Trade*. W. W. Norton and Company.

Rector, N. H. (1941). Drainage and Filling Methods for Mosquito and Malaria Control. *Symposium on Human Malaria: With Special Reference to North America and the Caribbean Region*. F. R. Moulton. Lancaster, PA. 15.

Rennie, J. (1991). "Birds of a Fever." *Scientific American* (July): 24-5.

Rennie, J. (1991). "Proteins 2, Malaria 0: Malaria Free Mice Offer Clues for Developing a Human Vaccine." *Scientific American* (July): 24-25.

Rensberger, B. (1992). Drug-Resistant Malaria Emerges in Cambodia. *Washington Post*. Washington (March 17) A4.

Reuters (2000). Mozambique: Money for Mines. *The New York Times*. New York (March 9) A12.

Richburg, K. B. (1990). Legend of Ho Chi Minh Trail. *The Seattle Times*. Seattle (May 8) B1.

Riley, E. (1995). "Malaria Vaccine Trials: SPf66 and All That." *Current Opinion in Immunology* 7: 612-616.

Rizzo (1989). "Unusual transmission of falciparum malaria in Italy," *Letter to the Editor, The Lancet*, March 11: 555-6

Roberto, R. (1993). Interview with Author. San Diego, CA.

Roberts, D. J., et al. (1992). Rapid Switching to Multiple Antigenic and Adhesive Phenotypes in Malaria. *Nature*: 689-692.

Roche Asian Research Foundation (1990). "Recommendations for Action and Research from a Symposium and Workshop on the Complications, Management and Prevention of Malaria." *Southeast Asian Journal of Tropical Medicine* 21: 498-512.

Rockefeller Foundation (1989). "The Health Transition Program: A Proposed Rockefeller Foundation Activity." New York.

Roitt, I. (1980). *Essential Immunology*. Oxford, Blackwell Scientific Publications.

Romeo, F. R. (1990). Interview with Author.

Rooth, I., et al. (1991). "A Study of Malaria Infection During the Acute Stage of Measles Infection." *Journal of Tropical Medicine and Hygiene* 94(3): 195-198.

Ross, R. (1923). *Memoirs*. New York, E. P. Dutton and Co.

Rougemont, A., et al. (1992). "When is Fever Malaria?" *The Lancet*: 690-91.

Rozendaal, J. A. (1990). "Epidemiology and Control of Malaria in Suriname."

Rukaria, R. M. (1992). "In Vivo and in Vitro Responses of Plasmodium Falciparum to Chloroquine in Pregnant Women in Kilifi District." *East African Medical Journal*: 306-310.

Rusell, R. C. (1987). "Survival of Insects in the Wheel Bays of Boeing 747B Aircraft on Flights Between Tropical and Temperate Airports." *Bulletin of the World Health Organization*: 659-662.

Russell, P. F. (1941). Naturalistic Methods of Malaria Control. *Symposium on Human Malaria: With Special Reference to North America and the Caribbean Region*. F. R. Moulton. Lancaster, PA: 347-52.

Russell, P. F. (1943). "Malaria and its Influence on World Health." *Bulletin of the New York Academy of Medicine* 19: 599-630.

Russell, P. F. (1952). "The Present Status of Malaria in the World." *American Journal of Tropical Medicine and Hygiene* 1: 111-123.

Sadik, N. (1988). "Population Pressure and the Medical Profession." *Tropical and Geographical Medicine* 40(July): S40-5.

Sadun, E. H. (1966). "Research in Malaria, Supplement to Military Medicine." *Official Journal of the Association of Military Surgeons of the United States* 131(9).

Salako, L. A., et al. (1990). "Malaria in Nigeria: A Revisit." *Annals of Tropical Medicine and Parasitology* 84(5): 435-45.

Sampaio, L. S. (1990). Interview with Author.

Sandoval, J. (1990). Interview with Author.

Sanger, D. E. (1999). "Clinton Widens Plan for Poor Debtor Nations." *The New York Times*(Sept. 30).

SarDesai, D. R. (1994). *Southeast Asia Past & Present*. Boulder , CO, Westview Press.

Satcher, D. (1996). "Renewal from the Viewpoint of the Centers for Disease Control." *World Health Forum* 17: 330-331.

Savitt, T. L., Ed. (1989). *Black Health on the Plantation: Masters, Slaves and Physicians*. Science and Medicine in the Old South. Baton Rouge, Louisiana State University Press.

Sawyer, D., and, Sawyer, Diana O. (1988). Community Participation in Malaria Control on the Amazon Frontier. Brazil.

Sawyer, D. (1990). Interview with Author.

Sazama, K. (1991). "Prevention of Transfusion-Transmitted Malaria: Is it Time to Revisit the Standards?" *Transfusion* 31: 786-88.

Scarponi, F. G. (1990). Interview with Author.

Schneider, K. (1990). Pesticide Makers Fight Export Club. *New York Times* (August 26).

Scholtens, R. G. (1972). "An Epidemiologic Examination of the Strategy of Malaria Eradication." *International Journal of Epidemiology* 1: 15-24.

Science News Letter (1944). DDT May Control Malaria. *Science News Letter* (December 30).

Science News Letter (1945). More DDT Victories. *Science News Letter*, (February 17).

Shanks, D., et al. (1991). Malaria as a Military Factor in Southeast Asia. *Military Medicine*. 156: 684-86.

Shaplen, R. (1986). *Bitter Victory*, Harper and Row.

Sharma, V. P., et al. (1982). Return of Malaria. *Nature*. 210.

Sharma, V. P., et al. (1986). Malaria Resurgence in India: A Clinical Study. *Social Science and Medicine*. 22: 835-86.

Sharma, V. P., and Kondrashin, A. V., Ed. (1991). *Forest Malaria in Southeast Asia (Proceedings of an Informal Consultation Meeting WHO/ MRC, 18-22 February 1991)*. New Delhi.

Shoumatoff, A. (1986). *The Rivers Amazon.* San Francisco, Sierra Club Books.

Shoumatoff, A. (1990). *The World is Burning: Murder in the Rain Forest.* Boston, Little Brown and Co.

Sikmmons, J. S. (1941). Transmission of Malaria by the Anopheles Mosquitoes of North America. *Symposium on Human Malaria: With Special Reference to North America and the Caribbean Region.* F. R. Moulton. Lancaster, PA, Science Press Printing Co.

Silva, K. T. (1991). Ayurveda: Malaria and the Indigenous Herbal Tradition in Sri Lanka. *Social Science and Medicine.* 33: 153-60.

Silveira, A. C. (1990). Interview with Author.

Simmons, J. S. (1939). "Malaria in Panama." *American Journal of Hygiene, Monographic Series* 13.

Simooya, O. O. (1991). "Severe Falciparum Malaria and the Acquired Immunodeficiency Syndrome (AIDS) in Zambia." *Annals of Tropical Medicine and Parasitology* 85(2): 269-70.

Sinden, R. E. (1991). "Still hope for a malaria vaccine ?" *Nature.* 349: 199.

Singh, J., et al. Case History of Malaria Vector Control Through the Application of Environmental Management in Malaysia. Geneva, *World Health Organization.*

Singh, J. A. (1935&1936). What Malaria Costs India: Nationally, Socially, and Economically.

Singh, K. (1976). "Malaria Control Means More Food." *World Health: A Magazine of WHO:* 34.

Sitwell, N. (1986). Malaria Returns: The Ancient Scourge Once Thought Conquered Now Threatens More People Than Ever. *Science Digest,* (July).

Slater, P. E. (1991). "Malaria in Israel: The Ethiopian Connection." *Israel Journal of Medicine Sciences* 27: 284-87.

Smith, D. C. (1976). "Quinine and Fever: The Development of the Effective Dosage." *Journal of the History of Medicine* 31: 343-67.

Smith, D. C., et al. (1985). "Laveran's Germ: The Reception and Use of a Medical Discovery." *American Journal of Tropical Medicine and Hygiene* 34(1): 2-20.

Smrkovski, L. L., et al. (1983). "Effect of Co-Irradiation on the Development and Immunogenicity of Plasmodium Berghei Sporozoites in Anopheles Stephensi Mosquitoes." *Annals of Tropical Medicine and Hygiene* 69(5): 814-17.

Smrkovski, L. L. (1984). "Studies of Resistance to Chloroquine, Quinine, Amodiaquine and Mefloquine among Philippine Strains of Plasmodium Falciparum." *Transactions of the Royal Society of Tropical Medicine and Hygiene* 78.

Smrkovski, L. L., Malaria Control Officer for U.S. Navy (1985). Interview with Author. Bethesda, MD.

Snow, R. W., et al. (1997). "Relation between severe malaria morbidity in children and level of Plasmodium falciparum transmission in Africa." *The Lancet* 349(June 7): 1650-5.

Sowunmi, A., et al. (1992). "Evaluation of the Relative Efficiency of Various Antimalaria Drugs in Nigerian Children under Five Years of Age Suffering from Acute Uncomplicated Falciparum Malaria." *Annals of Tropical Medicine and Parasitology* 86(1): 1-88.

Sowunmi, A., and, Oduola, A. M. J. (1996). "Efficacy of artemether in severe falciparum malaria in African children." *Acta Tropica* 61: 57-63.

Spencer, H. C. (1996). "Renewal Viewed from London." *World Health Forum* 17: 327-328.

Stanley, S. M. (1989). *Earth and Life Through Time.* New York, W. H. Freeman & Co.

Steffen, R. (1993). Mefloquine Compared with Other Malaria Chemoprophylactic Regimens in Tourists Visiting East Africa. *Lancet:* 1299-1303.

Stringer, C. B. and Andrews, P. (1988). Genetic and Fossil Evidence for the Origin of Modern Humans. *Science:* 1263-68.

Stromquist, W. G. (1935). "Malaria Control in the Tennessee Valley." *Civil Engineering* 5: 771-74.

Stromquist, W. G. (1941). "A Partnership in Malaria Control." *Southern Medical Journal* 34(8): 835-39.

Stroot, P. (1989). Malaria: Mosquitoes that Travel by Plane. *A Magazine of the World Health Organization*: 30.

Stubbs, T., et al. (1942). *Community Education for Malaria Control.* Richmond, VA.

Tadei, W. (1990). Interview with Author.

Tang, T. N., et al. (1985). *Vietcong Memoir*, Harcourt Brace Jovanovich Pub.

Tang, L.-H., et al. (1991). "Review: Malaria and its Control in the People's Republic of China." *Southeast Asian Journal of Tropical Medicine and Public Health* 22: 467-76.

Targett, G. A. T. (1995). "Malaria Vaccines-Now and the Future." *Transactions of The Royal Society of Tropical Medicine and Hygiene* 89: 585-587.

Taubes, G. (1997). "Salvation in a Snippet of DNA?" *Science* 278(5 December): 1711-1714.

Taubes, G. (1998). "Malarial Dreams." *Discover*(March).

Tauil, P. L. (1990). Interview with Author.

Taylor, T. (1988). Interview with Author.

Taylor-Robinson, A. W. (1997). "Immunoregulation of Malarial Infection: Balancing the Vices and Virtues." *International Journal for Parasitology* 28: 135-148.

The American Society of Tropical Medicine and Hygiene (1994, November 13-17). *Program and Abstracts of the 43rd Annual Meeting of The American Society of Tropical Medicine and Hygiene*, Cincinnati, OH.

Thomas, H. (1998). "Remember the Maine?" *The New York Review.* 10-12.

Tigertt, W. D. (1972). "The Malaria Problem: Past, Present and Future." *Archives of Internal Medicine* 129: 604-606.

Tigertt, W. D. (1990). Interview with Author. Washington, D.C.

Tizard, I. R. (1995). *Immunology, An Introduction,* Sunders College Publishing, Harcourt Brace College Publishers.

Trape, J.-F., et al. (1995). "Efficacy of SPf66 Vaccine Against *Plasmodium falciparum* Malaria in Children." *The Lancet* 345 (January 14): 134-135.

Trowers, E. A. (1992). A Nigerian Man with Fever and Abdominal Pain, (April 30).

TVA (1987). *Reservoir Ecology.*

U.S. General Accounting Office (1982). Malaria Control in Developing Countries: Where does it Stand? What is the U. S. Role?

Urban, B. C., et al. (1999). "*Plasmodium falciparum*-Infected Erythrocytes Modulate the Maturation of Dendritic Cells." *Nature* 400(1 July): 73-77.

USAID (1981). Anti-Malaria Project Mid-Term Evaluation. Washington, U.S. Agency for International Development.

USAID (1982). Bureau for Africa. Manual on Malaria Control in Primary Health Care in Africa. Washington, U.S.A. Agency for International Development.

USAID (1983). Workshop on Insect Control. Columbia, MD, U.S. Agency for International Development with Insect Control and Research, Inc.

USCDC (1990). "Transmission of *Plasmodium vivax* Malaria—San Diego County, California, 1988 and 1989." *MMWR* 39(6): 91-5.

USCDC (1991). Mosquito-Transmitted Malaria: California and Florida, 1990. San Diego, U.S. Centers for Disease Control.

Valero, M. V. (1993). Vaccination with SPf66, a Chemically Synthesized Vaccine, Against Plasmodium Falciparum Malaria in Columbia. *The Lancet.* 341: 705-710.

Van Den Ende, J. (1992). When is Fever Malaria? *The Lancet.* 339: 690.

Venediktov, D. (1998). "Alma-Ata and after." *World Health Forum* 19: 79-86.

Vreden, S. G., et al. (1991). "Phase I: Clinical Trial of a Recombinant Malaria Vaccine Consisting of the Circumsporozoite Repeat Region of Plasmodium Falciparum Coupled to Hepatitis B Surface Antigen." *American Journal of Tropical Medicine and Hygiene* 45 (Nov.): 533-8.

Waldir De Souza, M. (1990). Interview with Author.

Walter Reed Army Institute of Research (1990). Annual Report.

Warner, J. H. (1989). The Idea of Southern Medical Distinctiveness: Medical Knowledge and Practice in the Old South. *Science and Medicine in the Old South.* R. L. Numbers, and Savitt, Todd Lee. Baton Rouge, Louisiana State University Press.

Warner, M. H., Ed. (1989). *Public Health in the Old South.* Science and Medicine in the Old South. R.L. Numbers, and Savitt, Todd Lee. Baton Rouge, Louisiana State University Press.

Wasserstorm, R., et al. (1982). Malaria Resurgence. *Nature.* 299: 482.

Watson, R. B., et al. (1939). "Recent Advance in the Epidemiology of Malaria." *Southern Medical Journal* 32: 853-57.

Watson, R. B., and, Maher, Helen (1941). "An Evaluation of Mosquito-Proofing for Malaria Control Based on One Year's Observations." *American Journal Of Hygiene* 34: 86-94.

Watson, R. B., and, Maher, Helen (1941). "Further Observations on Mosquito-Proofing for Malaria Control." *American Journal of Hygiene* 34: 150-59.

White, N. J., et al. (1992). The Pathophysiology of Malaria. *Advances in Parasitology.* 31: 84-173.

White, N. J., et al. (1999). "Averting a Malaria Disaster." *The Lancet* 353 (June 5): 1965-67.

Wickramasinghe, M. B., et al. (1991). Forest Related Malaria in Sri Lanka and Prospects of its Control. *Forest Malaria in Southeast Asia (Proceedings of an Informal Consultation Meeting WHO/MRC, 18-22 February 1991).* V. P. Sharma, et al. New Delhi.

Williams, L. L. J. (1932). "Malaria Control and Anopheles Control Measures of the Past and Future." *Southern Medical Journal* 25 (6): 651-653.

Williams, L. L. J. (1939). "Malaria Prevention Activities." *Southern Medical Journal* 32: 851-862.

Williams, L. L. J. (1941). The Anti-Malaria Program in North America. *Symposium on Human Malaria: With Special Reference to North America and the Caribbean Region.* F. R. Moulton. Lancaster, PA, Science Press Printing Co. 15: 365-370.

Willocks, L. (1992). "Changing Patterns of Malaria in South-East Scotland: Implications for Practitioner Awareness and Prophylactic Advice." *Postgraduate Medical Journal* 68: 22-25.

Winters, R. A., et al. (1992). "Malaria the Mime Revisited: Fifteen More Years of Experience at a New York City Teaching Hospital." *Journal of the American Medical Association.*

Wiset, P. M. (1991). "Malaria in Travelers in Rhode Island: A Review of 26 Cases." *American Journal of Medicine* 91: 30-36.

Wojtczak, A. M. (1996). "The Need for Intersectoral Research." *World Health Forum* 17: 328-330.

Wolf, M. S. (1993). "Blood Levels of Organochlorine Residues and Risk of Breast Cancer." *Journal of National Cancer Institute* 85: 648-652.

World Bank (1993). Investing in Health, World Development Report 1993. Oxford, Oxford University Press.

World Bank (1998). The 'Better Health in Africa' Expert Panel. Washington, The World Bank.

World Health Organization (1987). World Health Statistical Quarterly. Geneva.

World Health Organization (1990). World Malaria Situation. Geneva.

World Health Organization (1990). Malaria, Present Situation of the Disease. Geneva: 11-15.

World Health Organization (1992). Entomological Field Techniques for Malaria Control. Geneva.

World Health Organization (1995). Vector Control for Malaria and Other Mosquito-Borne Diseases, Report of a WHO Study Group. Geneva.

World Health Organization (1996). Malaria, A Manual for Community Health Workers.

World Health Organization (1998). Roll Back Malaria, Fact Sheet. Geneva.

World Health Organization and UNICEF (1978). *Primary Health Care*. International Conference on Primary Health Care, Alma-Ata, USSR, 6-12 September 1978, World Health Organization.

Wyler, D. J. (1983). "Malaria- Resurgence, Resistance, and Research (Part I)." *New England Journal of Medicine* 308: 875-878.

Wyler, D. J. (1983). "Malaria- Resurgence, Resistance, and Research (Part II)." *New England Journal of Medicine* 308: 934-940.

Wyler, D. J. (1992). "Bark, Weed and Iron Chelator-Drugs for Malaria." *New England Journal of Medicine* 327(21): 1519-1521.

Yach, D. (1996). "Renewal of the health-for-all strategy." *World Health Forum* 17: 321-326.

Zabludoff, M. (1998). "A Great Killer." *Discover*(March): 8.

Zavala, F., et al. (1985). "Rationale for Development of a Synthetic Vaccine Against *Plasmodium falciparum* Malaria." *Science* 228(21 June): 1436-40.

Ziegler, K. (1999). "Why debt relief will not benefit poor." *BBC News Online*(June 3).

Zumla, A. (1992). Chloroquine and Proguanil Prophylaxis in Travelers to Kenya. *The Lancet*: 62-63.